THE PROGRESSIV
PARENT

KAVIN SENAPATHY

THE
PROGRESSIVE
PARENT

HARNESSING THE

POWER OF

SCIENCE AND

SOCIAL JUSTICE

TO RAISE

AWESOME KIDS

HANOVER
SQUARE
PRESS

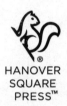

HANOVER
SQUARE
PRESS™

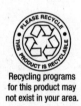

ISBN-13: 978-1-335-45506-2

The Progressive Parent

Hanover Square Press
22 Adelaide St. West, 41st Floor
Toronto, Ontario M5H 4E3, Canada
HanoverSqPress.com

Printed in U.S.A.

To my children, Asha and Jeevan,
who were born awesome.

THE PROGRESSIVE PARENT

Table Of Contents

1

the progressive parent's dilemma

I'm walking with my kids and their dad, Jesse, through downtown Madison, Wisconsin, the city I've called home for thirty-five years, coming to terms with everything I thought I stood for: justice, truth, and above all else, science, the arbiter of truth. Science brought my parents and me to Madison in 1987, the year I turned five. My father, who had been doing genome research in Washington, DC, at the National Institutes of Health, took a position at the University of Wisconsin. They packed up our bronze Pontiac LeMans, buckled me into the back seat, and headed west, where we would make our home in America's heartland. This city that's home to just over a quarter million people, the second-most populous in the state, made me who I am. What unmade me is something else entirely: parenthood.

My life's task has been to channel my *amma* and *appa*'s bravery. They left everything they knew when they came to the US from Tamil Nadu, the southernmost state in India, in 1980. Back then, they saw America as the land of opportunity, a font of innovation, a place of no limits, and they were going to see what they could do. Sprawled across the orangey-tan back seat on the road trip to Wisconsin, I felt perfectly safe. I didn't know I was en route to my demons and my eventual salvation.

On a typical, frigid Madison day in December of 1988, my baby sister arrived at Meriter Hospital on Madison's bustling Park Street, which runs north through several major intersections and ends at Lake Mendota. It didn't occur to us then that in 2011, my daughter would tear into the world in the same hospital, two generations arising in one spot half a world away from my own parents' roots. I lost my mind shortly after I gave birth, but science helped me find most of it again, just in time for my son's arrival in 2013.

At first, it seemed like my new fears were normal. After all, anyone faced with keeping a helpless creature alive and thriving goes through plenty of anxiety. It would be weird *not* to worry. But what I was going through was something else. In retrospect, I'm certain I've had obsessive-compulsive disorder (OCD) since I was a teen and that my first child's birth triggered an intense postpartum manifestation. Contrary to the common idea that postpartum depression is the main mental-health condition that occurs after someone gives birth, there are several in addition to depression and blues, including OCD, generalized anxiety, post-traumatic stress disorder, and psychosis. Postpartum OCD is characterized by vivid, frightening, and intrusive thoughts and repeated urges to perform ritualistic behaviors to appease those thoughts temporarily. My OCD's voice filled my head within days of a traumatic forceps birth, and it didn't like unadulterated joy.

Happiness comes with a price, my mind snarled. It was a price I would willingly pay. I had carried her in my body for this long, and it was up to me to prevent bad things from happening to her. I had to do everything right. I not only visually checked that the stove was off, OCD compelled me to touch the knob to make sure. I had to turn it on, turn it back off, and tap it five times in a row to ensure my senses hadn't deceived me and to keep the horrific visions of fire burning up my baby from materializing. It didn't matter that I'm a rational person. OCD had trained me to justify and compartmentalize the utterly absurd. *The potential for harm is everywhere*, OCD would remind me. It forced me to turn away from the light my daughter emanated and toward the dark and unfathomable chasm of my love for her.

Throughout the night, between bleary-eyed nursing sessions, I checked everything, layering my senses for added corroboration, touching her little chest with my hand, watching and counting her breaths to prevent death, and tapping the locks on our front door to prevent abduction, listening carefully to the sounds of the taps and noting the clicking of the bolt. I also felt compelled to seek information to make sure I was doing everything I could. The parenting books, internet forums, news outlets, warning labels on car seats and infant clothing, and well-meaning advice from all directions suggested that every choice could make or break her well-being. Like countless other new parents, I was led to believe that toxic chemicals lurked around every corner—in infant formula, the clothes on her back, the products in our home, and the foods she would soon eat.

Within a few months, I realized something wasn't right, talked with my doctor, and started taking an antidepressant, not yet comprehending that I had full-blown OCD in addition to generalized anxiety. The meds eased the worst of the terror and rituals, and soon, I found a beacon in the darkness: online communities of progressive, evidence-driven, science-minded parents helping each other parse through the information about birth, infant feeding, and parenthood. It snapped me out of the stupor of constant doubt and extreme worry. Part of me knew that I would probably always be anxious, but I couldn't keep reacting to my overblown feelings. I decided to fight my fears with evidence. I needed to know what could actually hurt my kids. Over the next two years, with the help of these science-minded parenting-community members, including veteran parents, intrepid scientists, and educators, I taught myself to read and make sense of peer-reviewed scientific literature in a way I never had before. Learning to understand the evidence or lack thereof behind scary claims was a desperate attempt at self-preservation. I relegated the worst of my demons to the margins in time for my son's arrival in 2013, and eventually, I found a good behavioral therapist who would diagnose me with OCD in 2014 and equip me with the tools to keep it at bay.

Learning to read the science to figure out if I needed to worry about the latest headlines was comforting. I felt like a new person, but I was left resentful of all of the fear-mongering targeted at parents, especially new mothers. Interacting with my peers made it clear that, on some level, parenthood is terrifying for everyone. Profiteers tap into this natural anxiety to scare parents about practically everything—we're talking epidural anesthesia during childbirth; chemicals in sunscreen, diapers, infant formula, fruits, and veggies; screen time; the flammability of children's clothing; the wrong kind of baby carrier and emotional attachment; the lifelong trauma of letting your baby cry for a few minutes; anything unnatural; and not gazing lovingly into your baby's eyes for most of their waking moments, to name a few. I soon learned that so much of what I thought would hurt them distracted me from what actually could. I channeled the resentment into blogging, intending to help worried parents make their way through all of the scary information. If science could help me, it could help anyone trying to navigate the fraught world of parenting.

When in doubt, or when I need to vent, I often turn to my fellow SciMoms, the founders of the since-disbanded nonprofit organization and blog that seeks to arm parents with the know-how to make evidence-based decisions. I launched it in 2018 with fellow science journalist Jenny Splitter, human geneticist Dr. Layla Katiraee, plant geneticist Dr. Anastasia Bodnar, and neuroscientist Dr. Alison Bernstein, all of whom have become like family. You see, even today, with decades of parenting experience between us, as scientists and science journalists, we still struggle to figure out what's best for our kids. We are lucky enough to rely on one another as sounding boards and as part of the extended village it takes to raise them, keeping the spirit of SciMoms going after closing the organization in 2024.

When added to the task of parsing through the evidence on any parenting question, viewing that information through the lens of progressive family values can make the quest for answers even more daunting. **That's the crux of our dilemma: How do we seek answers about parenthood and parenting that take stock of all of our values and evidence?** A note about this book's use of the word *progressive* to describe parents: the term *progressive* in the United States has evolved since its inception. Over the last handful of years, surveys from the Pew Research Center have bolstered the view that there is significant heterogeneity among left-leaning American people who identify with progressive values. Many of us identify as nonreligious while others believe in God/gods. We can be single parents, part of traditional nuclear families, or have nontraditional parenting arrangements, including kids with three or more parental figures. Some of us may or may not identify with the term *progressive*. I've heard some say that it reminds them of faux progressives whose actions are performative rather than transformative. I understand this perspective. But it is, in some ways, the word that most broadly connects people who are holding this book in their hands.

To really boil down the values many progressive parents hold most dear, look no further than those quintessential American family spaces: its front lawns. Where there are neighborhoods with kids and progressive families who feel safe enough displaying it, the yard sign of the ages that proudly declares family values is peppered throughout the nation. It reads *In this house, we believe: Black Lives Matter, women's rights are human rights, no human is illegal, science is real, love is love, kindness is everything.* Three activists in my self-styled progressive hometown of Madison created the sign in 2016 following Trump's election, with its iconic rainbow all-caps sans-serif font on a black background designed to pop during the snowy, soot-gray winters. They had no idea it would go viral, both online and across neighborhoods in the US, from Austin, Texas, to South Orange, New Jersey. One of the women, a fellow parent who collaborated in launching the iconic sign, activist Jennifer Rosen Heinz, had complicated feelings about it from the beginning. It was right after Trump was elected, "and everybody's like, 'What are we going to do?'" she tells me over the phone in 2020. So the sign "became a very accessible form of activism" that started to signal safe spaces, like when someone's car breaks down, "they look around, and they see one house that has the sign, that's the house that they're going to knock on the door," she explains.

Ultimately, Rosen Heinz says that the sign "encapsulates values." That can be a good thing, but she adds that it also can be a form of "virtue signaling," in which people literally stake the claim *"I believe in all the right things, I believe in science, I have my NPR tote bag."* She explains that it "becomes a kind of shorthand rather than an example of having done work or continuing to engage in work. It becomes a symbol rather than an active process."

Nicki Vander Meulen, defense attorney, member of the MMSD school board, disability-rights advocate, and one of the first openly autistic school-board members in the United States, says, "It's easy to put up a sign" to show support. "The problem is, are you willing to actually fight for what it comes down to?"

I'm chatting with Vander Meulen over coffee in downtown Madison on a summer day in 2022 and say to her, "You and I share the penchant for being very direct in how we talk."

She nods. I ask her whether she thinks that others' inability to handle straight talk helps cement the status quo in some way. "One hundred percent. People aren't comfortable talking" about what's most important, which is necessary to ultimately make things better, she explains. I've heard the sentiment countless times from all kinds of people fighting for the rights of children. I get the feeling that learning to tolerate discomfort is crucial.

All of these feelings about the sign are valid. My feelings are this. It's true that, in some instances, parents who display a version of the sign are participating in a form of virtue signaling. But whether or not someone chooses to display it around their dwelling, there's power in its message for parents if we also act intentionally on these shared core values: science, truth, equity, and justice.

Together, the ideas that Black lives matter, that women's rights are human rights, that no human is illegal, and that love is love are about *intersectionality*, also known as *intersectional feminism*. The late Gloria Jean Watkins, the renowned author and feminist best known by the pseudonym bell hooks, famously wrote about intersectionality before there was a word for it in her 1981 book *Ain't I a Woman*, titled after Sojourner Truth's speech by the same name, about the impact of both racism and sexism on Black women. Civil-rights advocate and pioneering scholar Kimberlé Crenshaw later coined the term as a framework for understanding how elements of people's identities converge as layers of discrimination and privilege. There are multiple elements of advantage and disadvantage, like race, nationality, gender, sexuality, class, faith, disability, weight, and physical appearance, that can serve to either entitle or oppress in dynamic and complex ways. In response to earlier waves of feminism focused on white, middle-class, cisgender women, intersectionality broadens feminism to include, well, all other women and marginalized people. With it comes the view that none of us, including our children, can thrive until all of us, and all of our children, have the most expansive opportunities to do so.

The values on the sign are also about equity, which isn't the same as equality. While *equality* assumes that systems automatically treat everyone equally, *equity* acknowledges that systems were designed to benefit certain groups to the detriment of others. *Justice* is basically equity in action: it's when anything is equitable and accessible for all, and these conditions are maintained in the long term. As for *kindness,* on its surface, the idea that kindness is everything suggests that everyone should always be nice to one another. Benevolence and friendliness are wonderful things but can do a disservice when applied indiscriminately. We often hear that we're supposed to *be kind* because *everyone is fighting their own battles.*

This response resonates with me: *Why would I be kind? I will be brutal and relentless. And ride into battle by their side.* I first saw it in a comic from Dino Comics, and it stood out for the simple reason that, often, doing the right thing means upsetting some people.

Yes, progressive parents are largely heterogeneous. But what really connects us is our drive to seek evidence-based, context-aware worldviews that are informed by science whenever possible and applicable, and to seek our own children's well-being along with equity and justice in the world. The more I've oriented myself in this way, the more I've learned to appreciate people who care about not only our own kids and families but all of our human siblings and their children. Although America is known for its individualism, there is a growing faction of us who think more collectively and are trending toward solidarity and a mutual aid mindset.

A specific phenomenon helps explain what we're shifting away from. The tendency to blame individuals' dispositional attributes for their ostensible misdeeds instead of seeking an understanding of the situational and contextual drivers of those misdeeds is a cognitive bias that's referred to as the *correspondence bias* or the *fundamental attribution error (FAE)*, which seems to be learned and not innate. Think of, say, a parent on the playground looking at their phone and not paying attention to their kid, or a stranger cutting someone off in traffic. One way to react is to assume that these perceived misdeeds are a result of character flaws: the parent is selfish and careless, and the stranger is an asshole. Another approach is to wonder about the external factors that played a role in these transgressions. This could look like considering whether the parent has had an overwhelming morning, or supposing that maybe the driver had an emergency.

Some research suggests that this cognitive bias that leads people to blame individuals instead of circumstances and systems is more prevalent among those who are socialized into individualistic societies, like the United States. It also seems to be more common among people of high status. To me, working to overcome this bias feels like a way to practice kindness. When it comes to our kids' welfare, to truly understand the big picture, we need to take a step back and examine why children might have certain outcomes rather than chalk up a child's achievement or health to parenting skills or individual disposition. Striving to understand the structural elements that create undesirable outcomes instead of assuming that parents' failures are entirely to blame—and interrogating the misguided assumption that avoiding these failures will protect our kids from those outcomes—empowers us. Context-rich information serves as our guide.

At the heart of this book is the question of how to take stock of our values as we make decisions about our kids' well-being while also imparting these ideals as they grow up. How do we go about honoring our families' unique identities while incorporating progressive family values and science-based worldviews?

However you slice us—we are certainly not a monolith—science, equity, and justice are our shared values, the ones that link us together no matter what we might feel about certain issues, no matter where we are in our journeys of learning, knowing better, and doing better. We are parents (and the other members of the villages who raise children) who strive not only to raise our kids in science-based, justice-driven ways but also to apply these values to the stewardship of our communities today and into our children's adult lives.

Though this is not primarily an anti-capitalist book, it will reflect some of what I've learned about how capitalism is not good for kids. I once believed in the pervasive narrative that the existence of extreme poverty was the natural order of things and that gumption breeds generational wellness while a lack of hard work causes suffering. It was a hateful view that I've come to see as violent, but it's common largely because it seems far more benign and logical than it is. In this false narrative, prior to the nineteenth century, extreme poverty among some of the population was an innate fixture until capitalism, and science, technology, and economic growth under capitalism, brought forth a consistent improvement in human welfare. This is a narrative popularized by powerful people, including Bill Gates and best-selling author Steven Pinker. In recent years, a set of graphs have spread on social media that purport to show the vast improvement of the human condition over the last two centuries. Developed by economist Max Roser for the online publication *Our World in Data*, it shows a significant decrease in child mortality and the percentage of humans living in extreme poverty and a hefty increase in vaccination, basic education, and literacy that corresponds with the rise of capitalism.

But the narrative lacks key context and "couldn't be more wrong" writes economic anthropologist Jason Hickel, whose research focuses on inequity and global political economy, in *The Guardian* in 2019. In 2023, he coauthored an analysis of capitalism and extreme poverty since the sixteenth century in the journal *World Development*. It explains that graphs like the ones Bill Gates tweeted have "several empirical problems," including that it relies heavily on GDP data, which doesn't accurately account for "non-commodity forms of provisioning" like subsistence farming, foraging, and access to shared resources. Colonialism and capitalism upended local ways of mutual aid and livelihood as they spread.

One of the most fatal flaws in this prevailing view is the starting date of the graphs Pinker used to back his claims that "industrial capitalism launched the Great Escape from universal poverty in the 19th century." The global capitalist economy was established in the late fifteenth and early sixteenth centuries, so starting in 1820 omits three centuries of relevant history, the 2023 article points out. "During this period, economic growth in Western Europe depended on processes of dispossession that caused major social dislocation," like mass enslavement and colonization. "The graph excludes this history and gives the impression of poverty in 1820 as a primordial condition."

In a nutshell, capitalism on the heels of colonialism created extreme poverty in places where it was previously rare. Extreme poverty isn't the natural human condition at all. The relatively recent improvements in human welfare coincide with the rise of anticolonial and socialist political movements. Colonization and its capitalist machinery are two of destitution's central culprits.

"If one starts from the assumption that extreme poverty is the natural state of humanity, then it may appear as good news that only a fraction of the global population lives in extreme poverty today" write Hickel and his coauthor. "However, if extreme poverty is a sign of severe social dislocation," then "it should concern us that—despite many instances of progress since the middle of the 20th century—such dislocation remains so prevalent under contemporary capitalism."

The 2023 analysis in *World Development* adds important context to another widespread, incomplete, and misleading narrative: that average human height has increased thanks to industrialization and the associated improvements in nutrition. In this view, the population-wide increase in height proves that human welfare has also increased from a substandard species-wide default. Here, too, the start date of this narrative is misleading. When zooming out to include those three omitted centuries, in many places in the world, the data show a drop in human height with the beginning of capitalism, followed by a relatively recent recovery in height on the heels of movements that bring about social change.

Instead of believing that capitalism provides for children like mine to live in abundance, I see that my own kids live in abundance largely because of their many forms of privilege. Ongoing systemic oppression keeps too many children in our communities from comfortable and safe homes in safe neighborhoods, plenty of tasty and nutritious foods, high-speed internet, recreation, and regular visits to good doctors. Whether someone believes that capitalism must be abolished or that it can be repaired, those who believe in justice and equity can agree that kids who are food- and housing-insecure aren't in this predicament because their parents aren't industrious enough. I like nice things, I believe everyone should have them, and I consider myself a fervent accomplice in the fight to take back the means of production.

We can also agree as progressive parents that, in America, we are all on stolen land living in a society built on the labor of the enslaved and the oppressed. As I write this manuscript, my family and I occupy ancestral Ho-Chunk land in south central Wisconsin, a place its nation has called Teejop since the dawn of time. In an 1832 treaty, the Ho-Chunk were forced to relinquish it. Decades of genocide by the federal and state governments followed, during which they unsuccessfully sought to wipe the Ho-Chunk from the state. I recognize and honor their legacy and resilience.

For nearly all first-time parents, the information we take in during the early days, weeks, and months can be overwhelming. During my pregnancy, a dear family member gave me a copy of the best-selling *The Baby Book.* Widely touted as America's "baby bible," with a cover featuring adorable infants of different races, it contains the wisdom of three MDs and a nurse. On its surface, it seemed like a progressive, science-based reference. As my pregnancy neared its end, I was reassured to know that we had this supposedly encyclopedic guide on hand. Babies don't come with instruction manuals, so this seemed like the next-best thing.

A few days after we returned from the hospital on a frigid January morning in 2011 with our newborn, as I fumbled through the sleepless nights that oozed into the exhaustion-frenzied days, I turned desperately to this thick, ostensibly authoritative manual to a child's first two years. As I paged through it, I learned that the choices moms make during this important time set the stage for kids' well-being for life. At the top of that list of choices is making sure to form a secure "attachment" between mother and newborn, creating a "biological pair." According to the book, babies have innate "attachment-promoting behaviors" that are so irresistible they "draw the parent to the baby" in ways that are "so penetrating it must be heard." As someone who believes in science, albeit vaguely so at that time, the language in the book convinced me that the Searses' advice was solid. Among the "seven baby Bs of attachment parenting" is breastfeeding. "The benefits of breastfeeding in enhancing the baby's health and development are enormous," I read, and there are also "magnificent effects of breastfeeding on the mother."

Whenever your baby latches on to your nipples, the hormones prolactin and oxytocin enter your system, and these "'mothering hormones' help form the basis for what is called mother's intuition," the authors wrote. Moreover, "the same hormones that help make milk make mothering easier," and "studies show that breastfed babies turn out to be smarter children." Another of the seven Bs is "belief in the signal value of your baby's cries." Here, the authors announce that they will "get a bit technical for a minute." *Ooh, science*, I thought. According to the Sears family authors, if one were to attach blood-flow measuring instruments to the breasts, "[w]hen mother heard her baby cry, the blood flow to her breasts would increase, accompanied by an overwhelming urge to pick up and comfort her baby." In essence, a "baby's cry is powerful language designed for the survival and development of the baby and the responsiveness of the parents. Respond to it."

I felt obligated to follow the science as per *The Baby Book*. If the science shows that babies who are breastfed on demand and picked up, held, and worn in a sling most of the time—babywearing is another of the seven Bs—develop better and end up smarter, healthier, and more successful, then that's what I would do. In those sleep-deprived moments that stretched into lifetimes, I ruminated on this overwhelming responsibility I'd just taken on. Within days, OCD quietly crept into those moments. The *O* in OCD is for *obsessive thoughts*. These can take infinite forms in people with the disorder—statistically speaking, if you don't have OCD yourself, you know someone who does—but they are basically vivid ideations of someone's worst fears coming true. At the time, among my most disturbing repetitive obsessive thoughts was of falling asleep and waking up to find that my baby had stopped breathing. It would be all my fault, and as I approached her crib to find her cold and lifeless, I would scream, and I would collapse. In the aftermath, everyone would blame me, too. After all, I am her *mother*. So I did what

OCD compelled me to do (compulsive behaviors are the *C* in OCD): I had to make sure that she would continue to breathe. What I craved—what all people with OCD, and on some level all people, and especially all parents, crave—was certainty. I needed to know for sure that I was doing everything I possibly could to prevent my terrifying thoughts from manifesting in real life. Next to my rocking chair where I breastfed and pumped around the clock sat my copy of *The Baby Book*.

I feel compassion for that version of me. I wish I could give her a hug and tell her that they would be just fine. I wish I could tell her that she would find her identity again. That there was nothing wrong with her as a mother. That practices like baby-wearing are fine and even ideal choices for some people, but they won't make or break a baby's lifelong wellness and success, and you don't have to do any of them. But in those first weeks, there was nothing anyone could say, not even my always-supportive spouse Jesse, to stop my constant hypervigilance.

Beyond a few basic parenting tips, more fundamental questions underlie this book. What can parenting accomplish? And outside of where we have tangible leverage as parents, is everything else we believe we have to do, from cooking from scratch to avoiding screen time, distracting us from living up to our values? When we stop seeing each and every individual parenting decision as paramount, will we take a deep breath, look up, and see others just like us and realize that we're in this together? What could we do with that communal power?

Some of those reading this book are in positions of influence, not only within your own families and communities but by virtue of your professional or other roles. As you read on, you may feel the urge to do whatever your position of privilege allows you to do in relative safety in any unjust situation. The concept of positionality refers to how social position and power dynamics shape people's identities, access to resources, and worldviews. Scholars, educators, and others have increasingly been considering how their own positionality affects their work. I think that the work of parenthood can also benefit from each of us reflecting on and staying cognizant and open about our own positions of privilege. Some people use social-identity wheels or maps that are readily available on the internet with the goal of gaining a clearer picture of how elements of personal and social identity overlap and interact. Despite some of my marginalized identities (I'm an atheist child of immigrants with non-European accents), I've spent over a decade learning to recognize and account for my unearned privileges, and we've tried our best to bring a keen awareness of these identities to our children. Having an American passport has given me an unearned advantage compared to those who aren't legal permanent residents or citizens of the nations where they reside. Though my skin color has been a barrier, having a light-to-medium skin shade in the beautiful range of skin tones in my large extended family has conferred a form of privilege in a world where colorism is still prevalent. Though my ancestors were colonized and subjugated, I never take for granted being able to trace my ancestry back several generations. Though my children have a white father, which grants them some privilege, he is also Jewish, which adds another complex dimension to their identities.

Nobody is born understanding any of this. It's okay to make mistakes. As someone who strives to honor my identity, I can assure you that there is no shame in privilege. When someone recognizes their forms of privilege, they are not necessarily accepting a moral reprimand for the relative lack of difficulty in life. The only shame is in willfully ignoring and hoarding it, and failing to pay privilege forward. Learning to recognize our own intersecting layers of identities can be deeply rewarding, albeit challenging, and a gift to our children as they grow.

How does a parent instill progressive values in our children, who are literally the future, prepare them to take the mantle, and ensure that the Earth and society will be everything they deserve? Obviously, this is a huge question and one that I have a few, but not nearly all, of the answers to. Ultimately, the aim is to steer away from progressivism as the type of ideology that lives on a 26-word yard sign and toward progressivism as a necessarily nuanced approach to the complexities of life. And there's nothing more complicated than parenthood.

2

healthy scrutiny of science

As we raise the next generation, one of the beliefs on the yard sign is not like the others: *science is real*. Does believing in science mean believing in its findings on issues that matter to someone, like that climate change is real or that our planet is roughly spherical? If so, I'm right there with the believers. Believing in science informs how we make medical decisions and choices about our consumption as parents, the foods we feed our kids, and the actions we take in our communities. It shapes our worldviews and the legislation our governments enact.

It can seem like a vast swathe of Americans doesn't believe in science, but polls show that most people do believe that scientific findings based on systematic observations are an actual thing that helps us discern the truth. **In fighting against those who proudly flout science and its most undeniable findings—a loud minority—we have glossed over the science that dehumanizes, justifies the displacement of the onus to individuals to solve systemic problems, and cements the status**

quo. The shaping of the trajectory of science by those in power has real effects on our children's well-being. To level up as progressive parents, we need to take a step back and learn how to scrutinize science in addition to harnessing it.

While researching for this book, I heard from nearly a hundred US-based parents who care about science and social justice and shared their views on navigating parenthood. For several, believing in science comes with trust. One shared that believing in science is about "trusting the evidence gathered in repeatable, comprehensive scientific research." Others indicated that it means "trusting" the scientific community on any given parenting-related question. Trusting the scientific consensus was another important theme that emerged among parents. One parent in North Carolina with two teens shared that believing in science means "[u]nderstanding the scientific method and believing the consensus of the majority of scientists on major issues." When it comes to parenting and science, believing in science means "trying to follow the guidelines that follow the consensus," said a parent of two based in Texas.

Science "does have some benefit if it's used correctly," says Victor Lopez-Carmen (known as Waokiya Mani in the Dakota language and Machil in the Yaqui language), a Harvard Medical School student set to graduate in 2024, cochair of the UN Indigenous Youth Caucus, and advocate who fights for the rights of Indigenous peoples, especially children. He stresses that the word *peoples* represents the heterogeneity of "peoples from every single race all around the world," not "just Native Americans," and the unique political status of Indigenous nations. For instance, in a 2019 study published in *Children and Youth Services Review*, Lopez-Carmen and coauthors looked at data on improving mental health for Indigenous children in Canada, Australia, New Zealand, Norway, and the United States. These are all places where there was significant genocide by settler colonizers in recent centuries.

It's hard to separate the science that affects well-being from the US government's "betrayal" of marginalized communities, Lopez-Carmen tells me. Distrust of science is often "valid." There is an "illusion" that "if you follow the scientific process, if it's in a journal, if it's in a book, then it's done, and as an Indigenous person, I don't necessarily believe that. I always question it."

As it's presented in the media, a consensus seems like an agreement by the majority of scientists on any scientifically studied matter. But a consensus is actually "a confluence of the evidence," says Dr. Alison Bernstein. Consensus is not the result of putting "a bunch of scientists in a room to conduct a poll."

Science is iterative, and when the body of that data begins to point to what looks like the objective truth, it forms a consensus. It is a living, breathing orb that builds upon itself, imbibing wisps of new knowledge and sloughing off that which no longer rings true. Consensus can be clear and practically unequivocal—think gravity, evolution, or the carcinogenicity of cigarette smoke.

But consensus can get buried by ideology and opinion, especially when a specific bias is held widely among the most influential experts in a given field. In scrutinizing science as parents, it's important to remember that, more often than not, the consensus on issues that affect children is more nuanced than it is with the shape of our planet.

We are taught that science is an unadulterated system and the worthiest ideas naturally rise to the top. But in the real world, science is only as good as its assumptions. And there are a lot of flawed assumptions in the science of children's well-being.

When it comes to parenthood, there is a slew of examples of how believing in science can help us. Believing in the science of germ theory means we turn to antibiotics when our kids have a bacterial infection. Believing in the science of climate change informs our consumption choices, our votes, and how we raise kids to be stewards of the Earth. Believing in the science that shows us that the Earth is not flat, and talking through the evidence that overwhelmingly supports that we inhabit a roughly spherical planet, can be a great case study in critically evaluating claims that seem bogus.

To believe that science is like the sun, which illuminates everything it reaches, is comforting. But science is more like a set of lanterns. Who controls the lanterns and chooses what to illuminate, from what angle, to whose benefit, and to what ends? How do problematic research questions and flawed findings around what matters to us impact our children? **When biased, poorly executed, wrongly interpreted, or irresponsibly applied science affects our kids, what, if anything, can we do about it?**

Science is another layer to scrutinize when facing any big question to which there are empirical answers, and there may be nothing more fraught with big questions than parenthood. In doing so, something closer to "science curiosity" than science literacy alone may be more valuable for parents. Research by Dan Kahan, a professor of psychology and law at Yale Law School, sheds light on the distinction between the two. In his 2017 paper on science curiosity and political information processing, Kahan and his coauthors look at why some people are more likely to engage in *politically motivated reasoning*—or the tendency to latch on to information that fits one's worldview and discard evidence that contradicts it. It's an important consideration because, for a democratic society to make the most of policy-relevant science, its people must have the capacity to recognize the body of evidence about any science-related question. The individual differences between who "is most vulnerable to the tendency to selectively attend to information in patterns that reflect their commitment to ideologically and like-defined groups, and who is the least vulnerable" is considered "the final frontier that scholars have yet to fully chart." Until recently, individuals with *civic scientific literacy,* or the adequate understanding of scientific terms and concepts to grasp a news story about a scientific matter, were thought to be less prone to politically motivated reasoning.

Kahan's findings suggest the opposite. Science literacy on its own can contribute to polarization in society. In other words, those with a basic understanding and knowledge of science are likely to use it to bolster their existing worldviews and discard what doesn't suit their narrative, even when their narrative is inaccurate. People who are more educated tend to be better at arguing their position, even when they're wrong. This sounds a lot like what drives some of the powers that be who make decisions about our kids' well-being. *Science curiosity,* or an ingrained desire to seek out scientific information to satisfy curiosity, may prevent or protect against politically motivated reasoning. People who scored higher on the science-curiosity scale developed by the researchers were more likely to seek novel information, even when it contradicted their views. Or as Kahan and his co-authors put it in a 2019 publication, "Science curious people—those who enjoy consuming science-related information—are less likely to hold politically polarized views about contentious science."

How to instill science curiosity among individuals is still an open question for scholars studying politically motivated reasoning—there's no evidence-based boot camp to train people to be science-curious. It may be a somewhat innate quality. Whether curiosity is inherent or can be instilled, it seems worth striving to be curious.

As we learn to scrutinize science as progressive parents, we are not primarily scrutinizing "the scientific method" itself. Science as a method is widely held to be one of the top ways to ascertain the truth. A 2020 Pew research study found that "a 63% majority of Americans say the scientific method generally produces sound conclusions." Practically everyone with a public education in the US has learned about it from textbooks, yet it's hard to pin down exactly what *the* scientific method even is.

Ask a teenager what the scientific method is, and they may refer to flowcharts that often feature anywhere from four to ten or more steps. The bulk of these can be boiled down to a handful of components: hypothesis, experimentation, observation, analysis, rinse and repeat. The way science plays out in the real world, including the stuff published in peer-reviewed journals, is messier. Hypotheses can be misguided, experiments can be sloppy, and observations and analyses can be biased. There is a growing movement to expand the definition of the scientific method, including absorbing Indigenous knowledge. Indeed, some argue that the exclusivity of what is and isn't deemed to be "scientific" in its methodology is a construct of white supremacy.

It's clear that one of the big governing values that go hand in hand with the fight for equality is "believing in science." I strongly believe that anyone can learn how to apply healthy scrutiny of science as it intersects with the issues that affect children.

Consider food. Feeding our children is also among our most innate human instincts. We know that what we feed our children is crucial for their health because science tells us so. Let's start with the food of babyhood. Even for those of us who are past our own kids' infancy, parsing through the science of infant feeding arms us with key tools to apply this scrutiny for parenting at any age.

To science-minded pregnant folks, breastfeeding is at the top of the list of consensuses on what's good for babies. We're told that "exclusive breastfeeding," which means an infant receives only human milk for the first six months and nothing else, is how humans have always done it—or as the saying goes, it's the science-backed *biological norm*. With that view comes the idea that baby formula is harmful. We learn that Mother Nature herself designed human milk. Unlike formula, which costs up to two thousand dollars or more per year, breastfeeding is free, we're told during pregnancy.

Since the mid-1980s, the discourse has been increasingly dominated by the idea that exclusive breastfeeding (EBF) is "optimal" and "normative" after the data started to gel into a clear picture that breastfed babies fared better on the whole. A growing number of studies showed that breastfed infants tended to have better digestive and respiratory health and fewer infections, a lower short-term risk for chronic conditions like asthma, certain childhood cancers, and diabetes, and were more likely to have better long-term educational and professional attainment. Several studies linking breastfeeding with higher IQs and better overall life outcomes gained a stronghold in the collective parenting psyche.

To boil down these scientifically proven benefits, leading public-health organizations declared a mantra: *Breast Is Best.* In 1991, the World Health Organization (WHO) and UNICEF launched the global Baby-Friendly Hospital Initiative (BFHI) to increase breastfeeding rates worldwide.

The mantra's essence remains the same in the 2020s. Amid the US infant-formula shortage of 2022, the American Academy of Pediatrics (AAP) issued updated guidance. In addition to its previous recommendation that infants be exclusively breastfed for the first six months, it also recommends "continued breastfeeding" complementary to solid foods for two years or beyond. It affirmed that breastfeeding is "the normative [standard] for infant feeding and nutrition" and that the advantages make breastfeeding "a public health imperative." For additional justification, it highlighted its decades-long stance that "medical contraindications to breastfeeding are rare." These affirmed recommendations came on the heels of a widely covered 2016 study published in *The Lancet* that claimed that increasing breastfeeding rates worldwide could save over 800,000 children per year.

I'll certainly never forget learning the Breast Is Best man-

tra, and neither have several parents I've spoken with over the
years. As I started digging into the truth, first as we prepared to
add another child to our family and eventually as a journalist,
imagine my surprise when I realized that the touted scientific
consensus that Breast Is Best is wrong. Though recommendations from the AAP and the WHO are usually based on rigorous evaluations of science, their stance that practically all parents
who give birth should EBF for six months is an exception. It's
based on the flawed application of spurious interpretations of imperfect science. Dr. Christie del Castillo-Hegyi, an emergency-
medicine physician, mom, and cofounder of the Fed Is Best Foundation, which promotes safe infant feeding and raises awareness
of the harm of the prevailing Breast Is Best ideology, tells me
that when these "authority figures" say that "the single best way
to feed your baby is exclusive breastfeeding from birth," it becomes "very difficult to understand the nuances, the exaggera-
tions, and the risks of such a recommendation." Parents are not
getting "true informed consent about the risks and benefits of
all" options.

As George Orwell wrote in the dystopian 1949 novel *1984*,
and as the rock band Rage Against the Machine famously repeated in their 1999 classic "Testify," "who controls the past
controls the future and who controls the present controls the
past." It's no different when it comes to science. Like with loads
of other areas of scientific inquiry around kids' well-being, teasing out the truth about breast milk and formula requires some
history because history shapes science and how we apply its
findings.

In taking back control of the past about infant feeding, let's start
at the beginning. **Though we're told that exclusive breastfeeding is how it has always been done, the truth is that some
infants have always received substances in addition to or instead of milk from their own birth parent for nourishment**.

If someone died giving birth, their newborn might have received milk from a lactating family or community member or an employed or enslaved wet nurse. Since copious milk production takes up to two to five days or more to be established, especially in those giving birth for the first time, segments of newborns in different traditions around the world have been fed a supplement in the meantime. Substitutes for a birth parent's milk have never been rare. Research on cultures throughout history and around the world notes that infants have consumed animal milk, soups, or liquefied rice or bread due to tradition or necessity. Long ago, the safest substitute for a birth parent's own milk was wet nursing, or feeding by other lactating humans. Some caregivers turned to "dry nursing," or an infant suckling directly from the teat of a livestock animal.

In the Victorian era, artificial feeding with flat glass or clay bottles with long tubes and a nipple on the end, which allowed infants to feed themselves became fashionable. With brand names like "Little Cherub" and "Baby's Friend," these hard-to-clean products were breeding grounds for pathogens that sickened and killed children everywhere, eventually earning nicknames like "murder bottles" and "death bottles." Bottle designs improved through the nineteenth century. By 1912, the advent of rubber nipples, ice boxes, and the acceptance of germ theory improved sanitation, and bottle-feeding became far less deadly. Today, as long as it's done correctly, bottle-feeding is downright safe.

The fraught history around how we feed our kids is inextricably intertwined with the fraught history of control over our bodies. It's clear that infant feeding is an equity issue and that barriers to breastfeeding are real and disproportionately affect marginalized people. The fight for the rights of all lactating people still rages righteously. No matter how cherished our right to breastfeed our own children is, so is our right to an informed choice to feed our infants with or without our bodies. Breastfeeding can be amazing, and in some families and cultures, it's sacred. At the same time, adoptive and other parents who don't breastfeed are discriminated against. Those who can't provide human milk, many of whom are LGBTQ, report feeling cruel judgment and pressure to do so by any means.

Amanda, a dear friend of mine whose child is now in elementary school, recalls feeling this pressure after giving birth. She had undergone a double mastectomy years earlier following treatment for breast cancer. The breastfeeding-promotion culture hindered her making peace with using baby formula, so she contacted her local La Leche League (LLL), a global nonprofit organization that provides breastfeeding support, to see if they could help her track down donor human milk. Amanda tells me that she was not as aware then as she is today that the benefits of breast milk are often overstated. She explained in her message to the longtime leader of the Southern California and Southern Nevada LLL network that she would not be breastfeeding her newborn because she has "no breasts to breastfeed with."

The representative explained that LLL doesn't provide donor milk and included information on organizations that might. The reply also stated that it's possible to "still secrete milk" after a mastectomy and encouraged Amanda to "consult early" with a lactation consultant because it "never hurts" for those who have undergone mastectomies to try to lactate. That reply did not sit well with Amanda, who ended up exclusively formula-feeding her brilliant kid.

Lack of informed choice—or of any choice at all—has long been a ploy of capitalistic forces that seep into parenthood, and it's no different with the infant-feeding battleground. In a world in which people have been bought and sold as property, and in which our time and labor are commodified and our bodily autonomy withheld, it's not only the control of our uteri that's in the balance. It's always been the control of our mammaries, mouths, and other body parts, too. In the antebellum South, in addition to giving birth to babies born as property, enslaved lactating people were forced to nurse their enslavers' babies. The control of people's chests and pelvises has since shifted to industries, employers, and governments.

In 1971, with input from the AAP, the FDA issued minimum requirements for protein, fat, linoleic acid, and vitamins and minerals, launching an era of steady improvement of infant formula into nutrition that increasingly resembles human milk. But there weren't measures to prevent predatory marketing. The formula industry quickly targeted hospitals directly, and Nestlé and others started bringing formula into vulnerable populations around the world. In places where sanitation and refrigeration were still scarce, several reports accused these companies of employing so-called milk nurses, who promoted formula and doled out free samples.

Against this industrial backdrop, free samples could be seen as a form of violence. Lactation works on supply and demand. Removal of milk stimulates milk production. Once someone's milk supply dries up, it can be extremely difficult or even impossible to get it back unless they give birth again. As obvious as it seems to those who know a thing or two about lactation, this fact about how milk supply works is not a universal part of the so-called mother's intuition that legend says you're supposed to acquire when you give birth. As the majority of birthing people have done for generations, I gleaned my breastfeeding knowledge from educated and experienced people passing it down. I didn't know any of this until someone told me.

Nestlé's messaging didn't explain that milk production works on supply and demand. When human milk supplies dried up, those who couldn't afford or access formula were left with worse options, like feeding other unsafe substances or diluting formula with water, which can lead to failure to thrive and seizures due to electrolyte imbalance. A few damning pieces of journalism shined a light on the deadly scandal. The first major exposé was a pamphlet titled "The Baby Killer" by journalist Mike Muller, published by the London-based antipoverty charity War on Want in 1974. In 1981, the *New York Times* reported that "about five million feeding bottles—many of them gifts of the formula companies—were distributed each year during the late 1970s in India, Nigeria, Ethiopia, and the Philippines." The World Health Organization and UNICEF found that as many as a million deaths could be attributed to these predatory practices. As a worldwide boycott gained momentum, in 1981, the World Health Assembly enacted a resolution to keep formula-industry marketing out of birthing centers.

That brings us back to BFHI, which the WHO and UNICEF launched in 1991 to encourage and recognize hospitals and birthing centers that offer "an optimal level of care" for infant feeding with the goal of increasing breastfeeding everywhere. Framed around the "Ten Steps to Successful Breastfeeding" guidelines, which are designed to "increase breastfeeding initiation and duration," the initiative urges caregivers to give infants "no food or drink other than breast milk unless medically indicated" until the introduction of supplementary food at six months of age. The steps include supporting "mothers to recognize and respond to their infants' cues for feeding," often referred to as feeding "on demand" without "limits to feeding times."

Hospitals that implement these steps can earn an official Baby-Friendly hospital designation. The initiative has also shifted the culture of infant feeding in non-BFHI-designated facilities, online parenting forums, and other parenting spaces. In short, thanks to BFHI and the global effort that went with it, access to breastfeeding support increased, and breastfeeding rates went up, to the certain benefit of babies without access to safe formula and water.

But in pushing back against the death and destruction that unethical formula industry practices invoked, instead of encouraging informed choice and access to safe and healthy feeding options, BFHI and its proponents fell into the same trap of withholding crucial information. Rather than recognizing that the negative outcomes of formula feeding stem from complex causes—including a predatory formula industry and systemic global inequity—its leadership not only decided to convince lactating people that exclusive breastfeeding itself can make or break their child's lifelong health and success, it also decided to hold lactating people themselves entirely responsible for their babies' immediate and lifelong well-being. In doing so, the science has imbibed the faulty assumption that formula itself is the *cause of* adverse outcomes.

Just a handful of companies manufacture most of the infant formula sold in the US. The formula shortage of 2022 brought to light just how vulnerable the supply is. That year, an investigation into unsanitary conditions at a facility in Michigan after four infants became ill led to a voluntary recall of multiple formula brands and the closure of a large manufacturer. The FDA wasn't equipped to handle what one official has called a perfect storm of "systemic vulnerabilities." The FDA acknowledges its duty to strengthen its workforce and streamline its regulatory processes to prevent another formula shortage. The system is still vulnerable in the meantime. There's no doubt that the formula supply chain needs to change. But the solution to the fallouts of a vulnerable system shouldn't be to put the pressure on individuals to provide an exclusive human-milk diet to their infants. It should be to hold the governments and industries that impact babies' well-being accountable. Rather than dictate that marginalized people around the world EBF for six months, justice would look more like ensuring that everyone has the time and resources to breastfeed or use pumped milk, if they so choose, or safe water and a reliable supply of safe infant formula if human milk isn't an option.

You may have seen a variation of the In This House yard sign that includes additional beliefs, one of which is "Water Is Life"—the translation of the Lakota phrase *Mní Wičóni*. This was a rallying cry for the Standing Rock Sioux and their allies, who

waged a campaign against the construction of a $3.8 billion oil
pipeline that threatened sacred sites and fresh water. Water is,
indeed, life, and telling all birthing parents to exclusively breastfeed while neglecting access to safe water—with which to prepare formula, produce human milk, wash breast-pump parts,
and so much more—is a Band-Aid on a festering gash.

None of this is to say that breastfed infants don't fare better
than their formula-fed peers on a population level. They do.
And it's not to say that breast milk doesn't possess some amazing properties, from antibodies to stem cells to a unique microbiome. It does. But there's a lot more to it. For parents, fully
informed choices involve taking into account all of the relevant
science and context, not just the science that organizations with
agendas want us to know.

An important note: human milk has been shown to protect
extremely preterm newborns from sepsis and a life-threatening
bowel infection called necrotizing enterocolitis, which can cause
holes in intestinal walls. Since newborns born at 32 weeks' gestation and earlier have immature immune systems, human milk
can help prevent these complications. If the birthing parent can't
provide milk, pasteurized donor human milk, fortified with essential vitamins and minerals, may be recommended for these
premature infants.

In the last few weeks of pregnancy, antibodies from infections
and vaccines pass through the placenta to the fetus. Full-term
newborns born closer to 40 weeks' gestation have mature immune systems and the benefit of those antibodies from their birth
parent. That's why full-term babies whose caregivers have clean
water and plenty of safe formula do fine without human milk.

For full-term infants, even though breast milk contains some
amazing stuff, there just isn't evidence that it's the mechanism
behind superior short-term and long-term outcomes. There's a
pervasive narrative that "you're depriving your child of all of
these benefits" if someone decides to formula-feed even partially,

says Daniel Summers, MD, FAAP, a pediatrician who practices in the Boston area. "A lot of times there's this message that any formula at all is going to be detrimental," and this message is "not only scientifically unsupportable, it's emotionally very damaging," he tells me when I call him in July of 2022 to talk about infant feeding, vaccines, and sexuality and gender identity. The narrative is "unfair, it's untrue, and it's harmful," and he tries to "actively combat" it when he sees parents at those "very beginning well-baby checks."

At the heart of the matter is the question of whether it's really breast milk itself that causes all of these touted better outcomes, or something else entirely.

Health research on the effect of a specific behavior or intervention falls roughly into two categories: controlled experimental studies and observational studies. In experimental studies, also known as randomized-controlled trials, groups of people are randomly assigned to either receive or not receive an intervention. These are considered the gold standard for making causal inferences because the process of randomization allows researchers to minimize differences between the groups that may influence the studied outcome.

In observational studies, scientists look at groups of people in the real world who do one thing versus another, and they observe their outcomes. These types of studies find associations between practices like breastfeeding and diabetes or cognitive function, screen time and body weight, or antidepressant use in pregnancy and conditions like ADHD. Association or correlation do not equal causation. For instance, while some studies associate passive screen time with higher body fat, screen time itself is not shown to cause fat gain or retention. Rather, factors that tend to be linked with screen time, like lower physical activity, contribute to these outcomes. Observational studies can be useful in certain contexts, such as providing context to inform future hypotheses. But there are challenges with inferring causal relationships from nonexperimental data.

The bulk of the data showing that breastfed infants fare better is observational because researchers face logistical and ethical challenges to randomly assigning some infants, on a large-enough scale, to receive no breast milk while others receive only breast milk. With all observational data, pay attention to confounding factors or any third variable related to the supposed cause and measured effect. Think of a researcher who wants to look at the effect of coffee consumption on the development of heart disease. Those who consume more coffee may also be more likely to work stressful jobs or have sleep problems. If people who drink coffee are observed to have higher rates of heart disease, cigarette smoking, which has been highly associated with coffee drinking in the past, or sleep disruptions caused by caffeine intake are confounding variables because they could also contribute to the development of heart disease.

Formula is assumed to cause bad outcomes while human milk is assumed to cause good ones, but the association of breastfeeding with better outcomes is confounded by socioeconomic status and forms of privilege. Everything from parents' education and income to neighborhood quality is highly associated with breastfeeding in the United States.

In wealthier parts of the world, people who breastfeed tend to be more financially secure, have better access to health care, live in neighborhoods with fewer safety and health hazards, and have reliable co-parenting relationships. Those who are most likely to breastfeed—especially exclusively—are the folks with the most support and time to do so. Layla Katiraee has shared how she managed to feed her infant exclusively with her milk. When she returned to work after over three months of leave, she used a pricey pump that allowed her to pump efficiently, up to four times a day. Unlike many workplaces without accommodations, she used a dedicated nursing room with a recliner, refrigerator, and sink—on paid time.

That widely reported 2016 study in *The Lancet* that claimed that increasing breastfeeding rates worldwide could save the lives of 800,000 children per year is based on the same flawed assumption that exclusive breastfeeding causes better outcomes. Brooke Orosz, PhD, a professor of mathematics and statistics and the mother of a child who had to be rehospitalized for de-hydration due to insufficient breast milk intake, was stunned to learn that readmissions for nursing problems are common and that health authorities don't track, let alone penalize healthcare providers for them. Since then, she has used her knowledge of statistics to advocate for evidence-based feeding. One problem with the 2016 study is that "although the vast majority of those *hypothetical lost lives* are in poor countries, this study has been used as a club" to shame people into breastfeeding in wealthier countries, she writes in a 2017 article published on the FIBF website. "The biggest problem, however, is that the article assumes 'near-universal' exclusive breastfeeding." She points out that, "[w]hile it works for some individual babies, no one has ever made it work across an entire society, not without allowing a lot of babies to starve."

Sibling studies help tease out confounders in observational data because kids who grow up in the same family grow up in similar environments and have the same parents. In 2014, US researchers carried out a major study that looked at data on thousands of sets of siblings born since the 1980s and compared breastfed and formula-fed infants. When they compared kids from different families, breastfed babies had a lower incidence of asthma, obesity, and hyperactivity and higher reading and math comprehension than formula-fed babies. When comparing siblings who were breastfed to brothers or sisters who weren't, those differences became insignificant.

There has been one major randomized-controlled infant-feeding trial that was originally published in 2001 (with follow-ups published since): the Promotion of Breastfeeding Intervention Trial. Researchers didn't randomly assign groups of infants to receive formula or breast milk. Instead, they randomized 17,000 mothers in the Republic of Belarus to either receive or not receive an intervention of encouragement and support for breastfeeding. Breastfeeding rates were significantly higher in the group assigned the intervention. Researchers followed these kids into childhood and adolescence and found that both groups ended up with similar neurocognitive function and incidences of asthma and allergies, obesity, behavioral issues, and more.

Often, assuming that a parenting behavior causes an unwanted outcome simply because there is a positive correlation between the two upholds an inequitable status quo. With practically every aspect of kids' well-being, there's a tendency to place the onus on individual parents while absolving those in power for their role in negative outcomes. In this spurious narrative, we parents can avoid these outcomes if only we put forth sufficient effort.

It's easier to put an outsized onus on parents to "take control of their child's health" than solve more complex systemic problems that have significant impacts on our kids' well-being. Ensuring the right to breastfeed is crucial, but "if you want to talk about an outcome that I think would make a meaningful difference in pediatric outcomes," exclusive breastfeeding isn't high up on the list, says Summers. He would rather see support for "the actual logistical needs of all families" like safe, reliable, affordable housing, childcare, and transportation. "What I think is best is to have a fed baby," he says. "It's not good for the baby not to be getting nutrition when the baby needs it."

A harmful outcome of exclusive breastfeeding that is too often glossed over is complications of insufficient milk intake, especially in the days immediately following birth, before milk "comes in" (around one in three parents who give birth will have a delayed milk supply, which is more likely when lactating for the first time). The truth is that when there isn't enough breast milk, supplementing could make or break a baby's health. There's nothing else "in medicine where we would just allow that to happen without informing parents," del Castillo-Hegyi says. But leading breastfeeding-advocacy organizations suggest that newborns who nurse frequently will get enough milk and that a newborn doesn't need much milk in the first few days. That's what I was told. If only parents understood that this is misinformation masquerading as the science-backed truth.

Summers has seen too many new parents experience the emotional pain of what feels like failure combined with the physical pain from bringing a whole human into the world. "Pregnancy and childbirth are exhausting," Summers says. Giving new parents a narrative of failure when exclusive breastfeeding doesn't work out "compounds the risk" of postpartum mental-health issues. "I abjectly detest the designation Baby-Friendly Hospital," he says. "It very clearly implies that if you formula-feed a baby, it's baby-unfriendly by definition. I think that it is coercive, and I think that it is paternalistic." He points out that of course "it's great to encourage breastfeeding," and that many people want to EBF from the beginning. But nobody should "feel pressured into choosing it."

When I realized I was struggling that frigid January day after discharge from Meriter Hospital, the BFHI-accredited birthing center in Madison, I felt deeply guilty. The newborn I always wanted was here, so why was I craving time away from her? If it's only human nature for motherhood to bathe us in warm, fuzzy hormones that facilitate lactation and a healthy attachment, then what did my new agitation say about me? Everything seemed to suggest that good moms have a natural instinct to carry their babies all day and nurse at every whimper. But even though I loved to cuddle my Sweet Pea, as I soon started calling her, whispering it into her soft head on my shoulder, I *didn't want* to hold and feed her all the time.

I thought back to when I was told during birthing classes that my newborn would stay in the room with me in the maternity ward instead of staying in a separate newborn nursery. This 24/7 rooming-in, one of the BFHI's ten steps to successful breastfeeding, is meant to facilitate frequent feeding sessions. In the hours after giving birth, it was difficult to stand due to sheer exhaustion and the second-degree vaginal tears that I sustained during delivery. At night when my newborn cried like a tiny velociraptor from her plastic bassinet, I painstakingly hoisted myself from the hospital bed to a standing position to pick her up, carefully get back into bed, and nurse her.

Once we got home, gazing at my baby while breastfeeding was intensely beautiful at times. But it was painful in the beginning, and I was also contending with the reality of nursing as per BFHI's advice to do so on demand, which in practice meant feeding twelve or more times a day, for up to forty minutes at a time.

According to the birthing classes and the lactation consultants at Meriter, a baby's seemingly incessant cries for lengthy and frequent feeding sessions are normal. EBF proponents suggest that colostrum, which is the clear, golden substance produced in tiny volumes before someone's milk starts flowing, is plenty. This myth that newborns only need a few drops of milk can contribute to the undetected starvation of newborns.

In the worst cases, it can be fatal. In a September 2022 report published in the journal *Children*, del Castillo-Hegyi, Segrave-Daly, and coauthors describe the case of Landon Johnson, who was born full-term at a BFHI hospital in California in 2012. He weighed 7 lb., 7 oz. at birth and went into cardiac arrest at three days old due to infant dehydration and, after 19 days of life, passed away surrounded by his loving parents. As his mother Jillian has written, he cried "all of the time" unless he was latched onto her breast. Since the prevailing narrative was that this is normal, she began to nurse him constantly, assuming he was taking in enough. When baby Landon was discharged, he had lost over 9% of his body weight, which was within the 7–10% weight loss that's considered normal in the first few days of the life of an EBF newborn and is still accepted in many hospitals today.

But millions of parents aren't told that universal exclusive breastfeeding has never been normal. BFHI's culture of assuming that EBF newborns are taking in enough milk when latched onto the breast seems to be contributing to an increased incidence since the 1990s of hypernatremic dehydration in newborns, a form of dehydration associated with high sodium levels in the blood, explain the authors of the case study. The increase has coincided "with global efforts to increase rates of exclusive breastfeeding before hospital discharge."

Landon's outcome is rare. Most newborns who lose that much weight will not die, though many will have other consequences, including long-term effects on the brain or other vital organs. One basic way to prevent the harms of dangerous dehydration and underfeeding in newborns is to revise "current perceptions of normal vs. abnormal" newborn-feeding behavior, weight-loss percentages, and frequency of soiled diapers, write del Castillo-Hegyi and her coauthors. This includes flagging newborns who lose 5% or more of their body weight for closer evaluation. Parent education also needs revision, they explain. For instance, it's important to know about the possibility of insufficient feeding in an EBF newborn due to delayed onset of copious milk production. Essentially, milk can be easier for a worn-out newborn to remove from a bottle than from a lactating human directly. Sometimes, even with a proper latch, parents and health-care providers have observed that newborns can be too tired or lethargic to effectively stimulate and remove enough milk from the breast, which can contribute to the delay in copious milk production in a kind of vicious cycle.

Parents need to know the signs that a newborn is not getting enough milk, including continuous, high-pitched crying or consistently prolonged nursing sessions. And they should know that it's not only okay to supplement with formula, in some cases, as Landon's mother Jillian Johnson often says, "one bottle" could save a life.

Still, in 2011, I was convinced that exclusive breastfeeding was best. Determined to give it my all, I nursed all night in the darkened living room, bingeing hour after hour of television network VH1, with artists like Adele as my only companions. (Jesse had no parental leave at his then-new job, so I figured that I'd let him sleep since he wasn't lactating, anyway.) "Grenade" by Bruno Mars became the first of many music videos that my children and I would bond over. His voice coursed tensely through my body as I held her close, knowing that I would catch a grenade for her. If only I knew what Summers tells me now: "The amount of emotional freight that's attached" to breastfeeding "is grossly disproportionate to the benefit."

I felt like I had no choice. I believed that not exclusively breastfeeding would give my daughter a subpar start in life because that's what the science seemed to say. When we were discharged from the hospital on day three, she had lost about 9% of her body weight. Like Landon's mother, I was told that I should continue nursing frequently at home, and we'd assess her weight the following day. I was practically delirious from nursing around the clock when we strapped our tiny newborn into her car seat to take her to her doctor's appointment on day four. At that appointment, I was devastated when, with compassion in her eyes, our doctor informed us that our newborn had lost over 12% of her birth weight and recommended supplementing my nursing sessions with formula for a couple of days. She assured us that I could continue nursing and wean off formula in a few days once my milk fully came in. *But how could it be okay if exclusive breastfeeding is the science-backed gold standard? How could it be okay if formula-fed babies are scientifically shown to have worse outcomes?* I would later learn that this bewilderment is all too common. As I slunk wearily into Walgreens for infant formula, my first parenting failure hung above me.

Fortunately, my baby didn't have to be readmitted to the hospital, or worse. Despite contradicting the common advice that supplementation could ruin breastfeeding, our doctor was right. Following each breastfeeding session, Jesse topped her off with a bottle of formula which she sucked down voraciously, while I spent another twenty minutes removing drops of colostrum with an electric pump to further stimulate milk production. The ordeal of doing this around the clock for three days produced the desired effect. By the time she regained her body weight, I was making enough milk to satisfy her, and we stopped using formula. Though I felt trapped as her exclusive source of nourishment, I got into the groove of lactating and did so exclusively for another five months and continued to provide my milk in addition to solid food until she was around fifteen months old.

What I didn't know is that I could have saved us the strife of those early days and supplemented far sooner. Choosing formula instead of striving to EBF would have been fine. What I didn't know is that, for some infants, losing even 10% of their body weight can contribute to immediate and lifelong issues, and that the pressure I felt has been known to harm some parents' mental well-being in even worse ways, up to and including suicide. What I didn't know is that Breast Is Best is not a science-clad mantra. And what I didn't know is that, while EBF promotion is not an industry in and of itself (though there's certainly an industry around it, from breast pumps to lactation cookies and teas to human-milk analysis labs), the most influential in the Breast Is Best camp, including the World Health Organization and BFHI themselves, as well as academics whose research is based on the mantra, have also reaped substantial economic and political gains.

Summers agrees that there is a "lot of really exciting science" about the properties of human milk. But the pervasive idea that human milk "decreases the risk of this long litany of chronic diseases and certainly anything about IQ just makes me want to run into traffic."

One concept that all progressive parents must examine and delegitimize in their own minds is IQ, which stands for *intelligence quotient*. Over the past several decades, parenting discourse has suggested that everything from the maternal diet during pregnancy to breastfeeding to certain music to stimulating toys and activities to avoiding screen time can give kids an intelligence edge, leading to the best educational, professional, and economic attainment. I remember reading *Baby Einstein* books to our infants, hoping I was doing enough in addition to exclusive breastfeeding to maximize their intelligence. The types of toys and other products that claim to optimize kids' IQs have changed since then, but the message is the same—buy or do the most science-based things for your kids right from the start and you'll give them the best chances at giftedness.

But IQ testing itself is "tremendously fraught," Summers points out. There is a pervasive "idea that you can really find out a person's potential, academically and professionally, with this test or that test," and there is "this miasma around them of objectivity, which is such garbage."

IQ tests are not an unbiased gauge of broad intelligence. Rather, they measure performance on very specific tasks that require various forms of verbal, spatial, and logical reasoning. These include the ability to retain and repeat strings of digits that an examiner reads out loud, perform arithmetic described in word problems, determine similarities and differences between grouped items, and complete visual puzzles. Intelligence itself can't be measured by a test; no standardized test can capture the dynamic, diverse, and unfathomable brilliance commonly contained within human minds. IQ tests "are culturally, linguistically and economically biased against minoritized students," Donna Y. Ford, PhD, a distinguished professor at the Ohio State University who studies gifted education told *Discover Magazine* in 2020. There's a built-in classist bias in IQ tests. They use language and measure knowledge that are most familiar to white, middle-class children. "If these tests were not biased, we wouldn't have different IQ scores along racial and ethnic lines—but we do. It's an indication that there is something wrong with these tests."

Another flaw in IQ tests is that they are biased against people who either don't care for or aren't primed to perform well on the types of reasoning tasks that they measure. Some extremely intelligent people just have less patience and motivation for standardized tests, and test scores are sensitive to this. Note that all of the above is only an abridged list of flaws with IQ as a concept. (I do feel some satisfaction bursting the bubbles of those who brag about their kids' IQ. If that's you, I'm sorry. It's like ripping off a Band-Aid.)

Summers explains that he doesn't "have a compelling reason" to think that holding parents to the AAP's exclusive breastfeeding decree is "the right thing to do." He stresses repeatedly how much he disagrees that breastfeeding can translate to higher IQs. The "idea that whether or not you nurse your child is going to be the thing that helps them align a little square the right way" is "just absurd on its face to me," he vents. He shares that his own mom exclusively breastfed him, and she also "wanted to exclusively breastfeed my younger brother" but it didn't work out. "He got supplemented with formula, and I will promise you, he is absolutely as smart as I am if not demonstrably smarter. He has a PhD in electrical engineering and I can't even understand what he does," says Summers, laughing. If "optimizing your child" is the "parenting goal," then, especially for parents who are relatively privileged, "breastfeeding or not is not going to be the thing that decides between, like, Princeton and struggling to make ends meet," he tells me.

Because we are told that science shows that "medical contraindications" to exclusive breastfeeding are rare, millions of parents wonder what's wrong with us when exclusive breastfeeding is elusive. It's an example of how our drive to believe in science can lead us astray and how exercising healthy scrutiny can empower us. Some studies show that everything from breast surgery to polycystic ovarian syndrome to diabetes to chronic stress and far more can disrupt lactation, and together, these conditions are hardly uncommon. All of that aside, humans have the right to bodily autonomy and to choose whether or not to use their bodies to feed their newborns.

Parents should get to decide how to feed their newborns safely and sufficiently by whichever methods work for them—and, as the Fed Is Best Foundation puts it, "all babies deserve to be protected from hunger and thirst every single day of their lives." For full-term infants and those with access to safe water, breastfeeding, formula-feeding, or a combination of breast milk and formula are all fine choices.

Beware that hospitals often don't provide comprehensive education on infant feeding. As Ranjini (Rini) Ghosh, a PhD student in law and public policy at Northeastern University and a parent of two who studies infant-feeding policies, writes in a 2020 *SciMoms* guest post, when a parent has to figure out feeding a baby in any way other than directly from their mammary glands "at 2 in the morning, they often don't have reliable information on how to do it safely." The reality is, many lactating parents will need to express and store milk at some point because it's not always feasible to feed a newborn breast-to-mouth every time. It's up to parents to learn how to use a breast pump and prevent contamination of pumped human milk. "The lack of education" on anything but direct, exclusive breastfeeding also means that parents using pumps "haven't been advised about safe infant feeding with pumped milk," writes Ghosh. There are multiple studies that find high levels of contamination of breast milk collected by pumps. "The points of contamination include the nipple, unwashed or improperly washed hands, and improper washing of pumps and bottles." Parents also should have an idea of how to prepare, store, and handle formula safely and make sure their newborn is satiated. Ideally, you will have familiarized yourself with how to do all of the above before having a baby, because figuring it out when you need it will be a lot harder. Crying incessantly or being too lethargic to nurse strongly are among the red flags that an infant may need supplementation. Though the Breast Is Best mantra cherry-picks science to suggest that supplementation can ruin "the breastfeeding relationship," there is evidence that, for people who want to primarily or exclusively breastfeed, supplementing with formula, or pumping and feeding human milk, can actually help establish breastfeeding in the early days while preventing excessive weight loss.

Feeding on demand is never, ever worth feeding when you're extremely sleepy like I did. In retrospect, I'm thankful that I didn't fall asleep in the hospital bed or on the living room sofa with my baby. Too many parents report breastfeeding their newborns in the hospital bed and falling asleep from utter exhaustion: falling asleep in bed with an infant can be unsafe. If your birthing facility practices rooming-in and you feel like you need some uninterrupted sleep, insist that a nurse take care of your baby for a couple of two-to-three-hour blocks between feedings.

If you want to breastfeed exclusively, for straightforward guidance including what to do if you're struggling, check out Segrave-Daly's "How to Breastfeed During the First 2 Weeks of Life": https://www.nytimes.com/article/breastfeeding-newborn.html.

If you do end up using formula either partially or exclusively, remember that you have done nothing wrong, no matter the reasons for your choice. Making sure your baby is satiated and safe and that your own well-being is taken care of is good parenting, period.

The Facebook group Evidence-Based Feeding & Parenting: Formula, Breastfeeding & More is a community of over 30,000 formula-feeders and breastfeeders, including infant-feeding experts, that "recognizes unique individual and family needs in baby feeding." They believe that "any reason is a valid reason to safely keep your baby fed." Please agree to and abide by group rules upon joining: www.facebook.com/groups/evidencebasedfeeding

For CDC guidance on how to keep your breast pump clean: www.cdc.gov/hygiene/childcare/breast-pump.html

For CDC guidance on how to prepare and store formula: www.cdc.gov/nutrition/downloads/prepare-store-powered-infant-formula-508.pdf

Find more resources at fedisbest.org/resources-for-parents/

Ultimately, when it comes to feeding our children, a lifetime of eating a variety of nutrient-dense foods is what is actually shown to make a difference in health and other outcomes. After infant feeding, there's, well, everything else that affects our children. With a healthy scrutiny of science, a scientifically curious mindset, and our justice-based values in hand, next let's look at another so-called scientific declaration that happens around the time of birth—the declaration that everyone is born biologically male or female—and how it harms all children.

3

revealing the gender and sex lie

Amid a growing uproar around gender and sexual identity in early 2022, with transgender children's participation in sports and public-restroom use among the most visible flashpoints, an unsettling rumor began to spread in Wisconsin. The story goes that the Waunakee school district, which is about twenty miles north of Madison, implemented a so-called furry protocol for kids who allegedly identify as nonhuman animals. I first caught wind of it on Twitter and Facebook, and then I kept seeing and hearing from credulous people, including fellow progressive parents, who were concerned that some school children now believe that they are animals and are allowed to act like it. Word started spreading that not only were kids allowed to sit at their teachers' feet and "lick their paws" but schools were providing litter boxes for children to use in addition to regular bathrooms. Similar rumors popped up throughout the year around Wisconsin and in states across the US, like Connecticut, Maine, Vermont, and Michigan, and in parts of Canada. On March 23,

2022, Kandiss Taylor, then a candidate for Georgia governor, wrote in a since-deleted tweet, "The furry days are over when I'm governor. Public school is for academics, not fairy tales." A few days later, Nebraska State Senator Bruce Bostelman earnestly spread the tall tale on the senate floor, asking, "How is this sanitary?" Bostelman complained credulously about unverified stories of children being allowed to defecate on the floor, asking, "Nebraska Department of Education, what is going on? State Board of Education, what is going on?" Bostelman eventually apologized after learning that the kitty litter rumors had been debunked.

As of this writing, these rumors are still circulating despite a slew of swift and thorough debunkings, including more than one at the popular fact-checking website *Snopes.com*, which reported that "The Waunakee school district has not seen a wave of students identifying as cats, and they did not enforce any 'furry protocols' in order to deal with these alleged students."

What fact-checkers have been calling the "furry panic" is a manufactured backlash against the rights of transgender and gender-nonconforming children. It is an extrapolation of the old right-wing, homophobic, slippery-slope rhetoric: *If a man can marry a man, soon we'll have humans marrying horses.* In the same vein, at the root of the kitty-litter-in-schools rumor is the bigoted notion that if children can be any gender or use the bathroom of their choice, what's stopping them from identifying as canines or demanding a dedicated fire hydrant?

Though they might seem benign in comparison, these rumors are no less wrongheaded than the old idea that interracial relationships are comparable to bestiality, says Ali Muldrow, board president of the Madison Metropolitan School District (MMSD), coexecutive director of the Wisconsin Gay Straight Alliance for Schools (GSAFE), and a mother of three. "It's a sensationalized idea" that is "just about getting people to associate what it is to be LGBTQ with something absurd," she tells me during one of our regular chats. Ultimately, forcing school districts to enforce the gender binary is "violent," she says. "For so long, kids who are gender nonconforming, who are trans, who are members of the LGBTQ community have been tortured." If schools "are not welcoming to our LGBTQ students, then they become dangerous."

Wisconsin is a precedent-setting battleground. As of this writing, MMSD's policy supporting transgender, nonbinary, and gender-expansive youth is one focal point of this fight. Defense attorney Nicki Vander Meulen says she finds the misguided political action the rumor has stoked "terrifying." She points to *John Doe et al v. Madison Metropolitan School District*, a parental-rights case filed in February of 2020, in which anonymous plaintiffs allege that district policy supporting trans and other gender-nonconforming children violates parents' right to "direct the upbringing and care of their children." MMSD policy prevents staff from disclosing personal information like a child's gender identity or sexual orientation to unsupportive parents because doing so "can pose imminent safety risks, such as losing family support and housing." The plaintiffs argue that, if any of their children were to stray from their assigned gender, they would need the opportunity to provide "professional assistance" to "pursue a treatment approach" to help them "learn to embrace their biological sex."

"Disclosure to unsupportive or hostile parents has high potential to do serious harm to students' mental and possibly physical health, including in some cases even loss of life," says pediatrician Daniel Summers. "I cannot overstate my opposition to policies mandating disclosure" to parents by schools.

In July of 2022, the Wisconsin Supreme Court ruled that the parents suing the district cannot be anonymous and must share their names with opposing attorneys. On a call on November 2, 2022, leading up to the general election the following week, Vander Meulen warns that the case is only "dormant" and that the plaintiffs will "probably refile," especially if "the right-wing wins." What's especially "scary" is that it's "still a terrifying template" for the rest of America, she says.

It's not just Wisconsin. This movement has been working across America to restrict rights for children and adults, fueling hateful rhetoric, book bannings, challenges to evidence-based sex-education curricula, and bigoted legislation. This "political moment" comes amid a long history of violence against LGBTQ youth and individuals, Muldrow tells me. Non-white LGBTQ youth are even more vulnerable. Queer kids say that adults are often the perpetrators of hatred against LGBTQ youth. **There's a generational divide in how we think about gender and sex, so it's up to adults, especially parents, to dismantle our flawed ideologies before we can truly protect and advocate for our kids.**

The notion that fostering an environment in which kids feel safe being trans or gender-nonconforming will "turn" kids trans or gay goes hand in hand with the equally fallacious idea that teaching kids about gender and sexuality is a tacit endorsement that they have sex as minors. In 2022, accusations of *grooming* have been increasingly weaponized against those who champion the rights of LGBTQ children. Anti-LGBTQ misuse of the term *grooming*, which is generally associated with sexual abuse, has its roots in the old, bigoted myth that gay people are pedophiles and child molesters. On April 19, 2022, the day after a Republican member of the Michigan State Senate accused Democratic Michigan state senator and mother Mallory McMorrow of being a pedophile and a groomer, McMorrow said in a speech that she "sat on it for a while, wondering, 'Why me?'" She explained that she realized eventually that opponents have weaponized the term *groomer* because parents who advocate for the rights of LGBTQ children are the "biggest threat" to the "hollow hateful scheme" of those who would prefer to discriminate against them in the name of "parents' rights."

There is no evidence that teaching kids about gender and

sexuality and making LGBTQ kids safer turns kids queer. "If you think that the existence of trans kids is sexualizing children…the problem is that you're sexualizing transness," as Sophie LaBelle, the artist behind *Assigned Male Comics*, which draws upon her experiences as a trans girl and woman, puts it. It's the evidence-based, justice-clad, context-driven view. Access to information and support allows children to grow into their authentic selves. Humans naturally develop a sense of gender identity before kindergarten. We all know someone who has dreamed of their wedding day or of having kids of their own since childhood. Kids often imagine what adulthood will be like, and that vision typically involves a gendered self. A child dreaming of a future in which they can be their most authentic self is the opposite of sordid. It's utterly ordinary.

You have probably heard the term *transphobia* used to describe deeply rooted negative ideas about transgender, nonbinary, and gender-nonconforming people. Psychologists have long used the suffix *-phobia* to describe an anxiety disorder involving an irrational and uncontrollable fear of and need to avoid certain situations (like heights or confined spaces) or things (like spiders or blood). But unlike, say, claustrophobia or arachnophobia, transphobia—like homophobia, Islamophobia, or xenophobia—is not a mental-health condition. Some antioppression advocates have pointed out that the term *transmisia* is more accurate because *misia* means *hatred*, which emphasizes the prejudice and bigotry that drives these views and resulting actions. While imperfect, the term *transphobia* can be useful largely because it's more widely recognized.

Here are a few definitions of terms used to talk about sex and gender:

Gender refers to socially constructed roles, behaviors, activities, or attributes that a given culture associates with being a woman, man, girl, or boy. It varies from culture to culture and is dynamic.

Sex is a biological category based on reproductive, anatomical, and genetic characteristics.

Sexuality or *sexual orientation* refers to feelings of romantic or sexual attraction. Examples include gay, lesbian, heterosexual, bisexual, pansexual, and asexual. Sexual orientation can be fluid, and people can have more than one. Sex, gender, and sexuality each exist on their own spectrums, though all three are related.

The *gender binary* is the fallacious idea that only two distinct genders exist. It also refers to the system of gender classification that only acknowledges two distinct categories of male or female.

Cisgender describes anyone whose gender aligns with their sex assigned at birth.

LGBTQ: The initialism, which stands for lesbian, gay, bisexual, transgender, and queer and has a rich history, has evolved to not only refer to homosexual, bisexual, and transgender folks, but anyone who isn't heterosexual or cisgender. The Q for *queer* was once used as a slur for homosexual people but has since been reclaimed by some to denote pride. It also refers to the emerging academic field of queer studies. The longer acronym LGBTQIA is often used to explicitly include intersex and asexual individuals.

Transgender, sometimes shortened to *trans*, is an umbrella term for those whose gender identity differs from their assigned sex at birth. It can refer to a binary gender that is "opposite" or "across from" the sex they were assigned at birth.

Nonbinary is a term for gender identity or expression that isn't solely girl/woman or boy/man.

Gender nonconforming is an umbrella term for someone who doesn't conform to a culture's traditional gender norms.

Some gender-nonconforming and nonbinary folks identify as transgender, some don't.

Genderqueer describes a person whose gender identity cannot be categorized as solely male or female.

Gender *dysphoria* is the experience of incongruence between someone's body, gender identity, and gender expression, which some—but not all—gender-nonconforming, trans, or nonbinary people experience.

Transitioning, which is also known as *gender affirmation* or *gender confirmation*, is when someone changes the way they dress, chooses a new name, modifies their mannerisms, leans into their gender in other ways, or gets help from a doctor to reach *congruence*, or a sense of comfort, harmony, or alignment between their body, identity, and expression. Transitioning can look like an obvious and drastic outward change or can be more subtle, with bigger shifts taking place on the inside, and everything in between. There is no one way to transition.

Transphobia also thrives on the left

Holding transphobic views and seeking to oppress gender-nonconforming children is not only a right-wing phenomenon. It is with this form of dehumanization that a sect of progressives aligns itself with the right wing. On April 23, 2022, at the Central branch of the Madison Public Library, a group of around a hundred self-professed trans-exclusionary radical feminists, or TERFs, convened for a weekend-long, "female-only" TERF conference. First popularized in 2008, the term *TERF* describes people who claim to be feminists but who deny that trans women and girls are "real" women and girls. While some consider TERF to be a slur and prefer to go by "gender critical" and some with these ideologies reject labels altogether, others proudly claim it, including members of the group convened at the library that day.

The leftists who hold these views support the rights of homosexuals but not of trans folks.

I headed downtown around one o'clock on that warm spring Saturday and joined the group of demonstrators outside the library who were protesting the TERF conference, bearing signs with slogans like *Transphobia Kills*. While the TERF-conference speakers made their statements inside the library, those protesting antitrans ideology chalked the sidewalk with words like *Protect Trans Kids*. When attendees of the "female-only" conference streamed out of the library to march to a scheduled rally on the front steps of the capitol building, protesters followed behind, shouting their opposing slogans. A few of the TERFs lingered, exchanging barbs with the counterprotesters. Among the most unsettling claims from TERF-conference attendees was that their side of the debate was the intellectual and scientific side.

Whether they call themselves TERFs, gender-critical, or something else, those who oppose the existence and validity of trans people are not being very scientific, says Vander Meulen. The truth is neither "quick" nor "easy," she tells me over coffee in the summer of 2022. Their ideology may appear benign and even seem to make sense. It wasn't long ago that it made sense to me. **In a nutshell, the lie of the gender and sex binaries is this: sex is immutable. Those born with XY chromosomes and penises will always be "biologically male" while babies with XX chromosomes and a vagina will always be "biologically female," and to say otherwise is denying the scientific facts.** I bought into this ideology as recently as the mid-2010s, not realizing that it's fundamentally hateful and pseudoscientific.

It's no coincidence that the most insidious, harmful bigotry can seem benign, reasonable, and yes, even *scientific*. We internalize it without dissonance. The binary has been drilled into us for so long that it can be grueling to dislodge.

Summers warns that these seemingly scientific arguments

around biology are dangerous because they provide "an intellectual-sounding justification for otherwise just frank bigotry." Many progressive parents seem to agree that, yeah, using people's pronouns is, of course, important. What many progressives get hung up on is the unexamined, wholesale acceptance that binary sex is an immutable, innate thing. A 2022 study of over 10,000 US adults from the Pew Research Center on Americans' views about gender identity suggests that this view is spreading.

In the mid-2010s, when my children were toddlers, I had begun to grapple with why so many seemingly science-minded people were adamant that it's wrong to say that kids who are born with XY chromosomes and penises are "biologically male." Though she had every right to tell me off for my dehumanizing questions, a trans researcher and fellow blogger with more patience than I deserved began to explain why I was so wrong. This exchange set me on a quest to understand the truth. Nearly a decade later, not only would I gain a deeper view of humanity, children, sex, and gender, I would realize that I have always been nonbinary, even though I have given birth to two babies. In retrospect, I did feel moderate dysphoria during pregnancy and soon after giving birth but am at relative ease now that I'm not hosting a human in my body or lactating. The idea of someone like me being anything but *female* would have been preposterous to me just years earlier.

It chills me to realize that, as benign and convincing as it seems on its surface, this mythology that gender and sex are binary, which is sometimes shortened to *binarism*, underlies not only discrimination against trans children but against all children. What we learned in the 1990s about sex and gender is about as real as that old frictionless plane in physics. Biology is "so much richer and more complex," Liza Brusman, a molecular biologist, neuroscientist, and PhD candidate in molecular, cellular, and developmental biology at the University of Colorado Boulder, tells me on a call in 2022. In addition to being harmful, "reducing sex into just two categories is not actually very accurate."

"This isn't just about trans kids," Muldrow explains. Transphobia leads to direct harm not only to transgender children but to everyone. With all of this gender-based legislation in the pipeline, Muldrow reminds me that "nobody should get to tell" people how to be who they are. It's the same ideology behind wanting to restrict abortion, she says.

Abortion isn't just about a "woman's" right to choose, it's about a person's right to choose. Tiffany Green, PhD, a mother of two and a professor in the departments of population health sciences and obstetrics and gynecology at the University of Wisconsin-Madison explains that, as a researcher, it initially felt unnatural to use gender-neutral language for birthing people. As we sit outdoors on a warm day in August 2022, she and I commiserate about feeling increasingly uneasy with the language around "women's right to choose."

"I struggled a little bit with 'pregnant people' because it feels awkward," Green says. "Anything outside of the gender binary is not comfortable," at least until you get used to it. As a researcher, accuracy eventually won out. Not only women get pregnant and give birth. Trans men, gender-nonconforming people with uteri, and yes, "adolescents have children," she says with exasperation.

What do trans rights have to do with the rights of all girls, let alone abortion? It comes down to *biological essentialism*, which is also known as biological determinism. It's the notion that life on Earth can be grouped into natural, hierarchical categories and that some humans fall into a norm while all others are abnormal or inferior. Biological essentialism is insidious. It seems benign and logical, but this fabrication is at the heart of inequity. Keira Havens, a US Air Force veteran, molecular biologist, activist, and writer based in Colorado, explained to me in

November 2022 that it was not merely made up but made up by "a guy who thought rocks could fuck," and "decided that you could read God's Divine Plan in the way the living world organized itself." She's referring to Carl Linnaeus, who's best known for formalizing the system of naming organisms that we use today. He also surmised that minerals could be classified based on sexual reproduction and hierarchy in the same way as animals and plants (so yeah, he seriously thought that rocks may be mating in a biological sense). Using his then-new taxonomic system, Linnaeus classified humans as belonging to the genus *Homo* and the species *sapiens*. Biological essentialism around race, for instance, is the assumption that race is a natural, genetic category and that people who are of the same race share many traits. He was obsessed with order and organization and described his contribution to science: "God created, but Linnaeus organized." (These guys have generally not been known for their humility.) But practically all life defies strict categorization.

Biological essentialism harms men and boys, too. It cements toxic masculinity or the idea that men and boys don't cry and are naturally aggressive. It's the glue that holds together the notion that men are inherently evil and predatory. It prevents boys from being their true selves.

A set of scientific and social constructs bolster the binary. How do we protect our children from discrimination based on sex and gender? To answer that question, we need an updated view of what science says about sex and gender. Scrutiny of so-called scientific arguments for gender and sex binarism reveals that, like the truth about infant feeding, the scientific truth about the binary is nothing like what we've been led to believe.

What even is a *male* or *female*? Before reading on, take a minute or two and, with nonjudgmental curiosity, ask yourself what comes to mind when you think of a male or a female human, and make note of it.

It's still common for people to use the terms *sex* and *gender* interchangeably, but they are not the same thing. When the distinction is made, it's often boiled down to the idea that gender is about someone's socialization, feelings, experience, and expression, while sex is about a person's biology. "Debates about sex are often framed falsely as scientific versus cultural arguments, whereby the former by virtue of being grounded in biology are seen as tied to nature and thus truth, whereas the latter are seen as hectoring from a postmodern gender La La Land," writes cultural anthropologist Katrina Karkazis in a 2019 article in *The Lancet*. This framing "profoundly misconstrues who is hewing to science." This is not about "science versus social constructionism as some argue; it's about the calculated use of 'biological sex' to buttress obsolete thinking about sex."

Gender is a "social construct," but Brusman warns against the tendency to assume that social constructs are "not real." When a concept is socially constructed, that means it exists because humans created and defined it. Like other social constructs, including national borders and money, gender "impacts people in very real, tangible ways," she says.

Researchers who study human biology are increasingly centering the fact that sex and gender are inextricably entangled throughout a lifetime. Rather than distinct categories with ostensibly little bearing on one another, gender and sex are connected. Gender norms influence traits that are associated with sex in a dynamic interaction. Another increasingly common framing is to acknowledge the complex relationship between not just the two categories of gender and sex, but three dimensions: 1) someone's body, 2) their identity, or internal experience, and 3) their social gender, which includes outward expression.

Living in a gendered society has biological impacts on the body. One example of this is bone density, which is traditionally thought to be higher on average in males. With this comes the belief that sex can be reliably determined from skeletal remains.

Only recently are we learning about the many gendered factors that influence bone density. In a 2022 article in *The International Journal of Environmental Research and Public Health*, Stacey Ritz, PhD, an associate professor of pathology and molecular medicine at McMaster University in Ontario, and coauthor Lorraine Greaves, a feminist and clinical professor at the Centre of Excellence for Women's Health at the University of British Columbia in Vancouver, write about the need to "transcend" the male and female binary in biomedical research. Their call for change isn't new. Scholars have been expressing this need for decades. Referring to a 2005 article on how culture shapes bones, Ritz and Greaves explain that since bones seem to be clearly biological and are affected by hormones, it has been tempting for scientists to attribute differences in bone density to sex. But there hasn't been evidence to suggest that females naturally have lower bone density, and lots of evidence that this difference doesn't hold up across populations. For instance, in communities in China where women traditionally work daily in the fields, bone density is higher on average in women than in men. The type, intensity, and frequency of weight-bearing activities in which an individual participates, dietary differences, alcohol consumption, and more have been shown to affect bone density. When viewing the bigger picture, the correlation of our constructed categories of *male* and *female* with bone density in white Americans has yet again led to a misguided assumption about causality. "A commitment to embracing complexity and dynamism will be necessary to push sex and gender science in biomedical research forward and to avoid furthering essentialism, determinism, and categorical thinking," write Ritz and Greaves. I'm convinced that the same commitment is crucial for progressive parents. Biomedical researchers are "on the cusp of a paradigm shift," in how they think about gender and sex, they write. I'm convinced that, as progressive parents, we're on the cusp of a paradigm shift, too.

To attempt to pin down the sometimes-nebulous distinction between *female* and *male*, some researchers refer to *3G sex*. This genotype-gonads-genitalia triad is a categorization system in which *female* = XX, ovaries, uterus, fallopian tubes, and a vulva, and *male* = XY, testes, prostate, seminal vesicles, scrotum, and penis.

Another possible definition of sex is based on the size of someone's sex cells. Testicles, ovaries, and all other parts aside, from an evolutionary perspective, the key distinction is whether an individual produces a few large eggs or millions of small sperm.

Scratch the surface and even those seemingly precise definitions fail to capture biological sex. In school, we often learn that X and Y chromosomes are responsible for sex determination, or the process by which developing animals become either male or female. Prior to the discovery of these sex chromosomes in the early twentieth century, there were hundreds of documented wrong ideas about how it works in humans. Aristotle, for instance, thought that male babies were a product of heat and dryness produced by particularly virile male partners during intercourse, while female babies were a product of an ineffectual male partner lacking sufficient heat. Seriously.

Around the turn of the twentieth century, a scientist by the name of Nettie Stevens was pursuing the right answer to sex determination. Her interest came on the heels of work by Gregor Mendel, the monk whose famous experiments in the 1860s used plant breeding to elucidate basic principles of inheritance of *traits*, or observable characteristics, in the common pea plant. People who took a high-school biology class may recall the Punnett squares used to predict the types of offspring in a crossbreeding experiment. I promise that I bring this up for a worthwhile reason, so please bear with me. In his experiments, Mendel figured out that some unknown substance, which we now know as DNA, passes traits from parents to offspring. In his plants—and with myriad traits across a slew of animals, plants, and other organisms, as scientists have learned since—the observable characteristics he studied, like yellow or green pea color or smooth or wrinkly pea skin, are inherited in predictable ways based on whether a trait is dominant or recessive. In these plants, the green *allele*, or a genetic variety of a specific trait, is dominant for the trait of color, and yellow is recessive. The green allele is denoted capital G to show dominance, and yellow is denoted with a lowercase *g*. Any plant that inherits at least one green allele, or either GG or Gg, will be green, while only plants that are gg will be yellow. Here, GG, Gg, and gg are all different *genotypes*, or individual pea plants' genetic makeups, and whether they're green or yellow are their *phenotype*, or the observable characteristics. There are lots of traits that are thought to be inherited in this Mendelian way—like hair color in some dogs, cleft chins and widow's peaks in humans, petal colors in some flowers, and more.

Inspired by Mendel, in 1905, Nettie Stevens made a breakthrough. Eggs and sperm come from a process called *meiosis*, in which a single cell divides twice to produce sex cells containing half the original amount of genetic information. By Stevens's time, chromosomes, or the threadlike structures in the nucleus of cells, were known to act as vectors of heredity. While looking at mealworm sperm and eggs through her microscope, she saw that half of the sperm had nine large chromosomes and one small one, and that the eggs all had ten large chromosomes. The cells of the bodies of male mealworms had nineteen large chromosomes and one small one, and cells from females had twenty large chromosomes. She concluded that this small chromosome, which we now know as the Y chromosome, must play a critical role in determining the sex of offspring.

Since then, we've learned just how variable sex determination actually is.

In the animal kingdom, there is a vast spectrum of ways to be either male, female, both, or neither. Some species have an environmental trigger to sex differentiation: you may have heard that in many egg-laying reptiles, the incubation temperature determines the sex of the offspring, a process known as temperature-dependent sex determination. Many of us are familiar with the XX and XY sex-determination system, which happens in humans, most mammals, and lots of insects like the mealworm.

But even in humans, sex and gender are far more than just XX or XY. They're not just traits inherited in the simplistic Mendelian way. We need to "move beyond Mendel," to combat both sexism and racism in society, says Brian Donovan, a senior science education researcher at the Humane Genetics Research Lab at the nonprofit BSCS Science Learning, headquartered in Colorado Springs, Colorado. The lab explores how biology education, especially in middle school and high school, can tackle racism and sexism in society. Their research suggests that the oversimplification of genetics and essentialist genetic constructs of race, sex, and gender in the curriculum can increase students' tendency toward both racist and sexist thinking. The researchers call this oversimplification "a big scary problem." Fortunately, they've elucidated an approach that significantly reduces this tendency, including a curriculum that focuses on "honoring the complexity of genetics." It allows students to develop a more nuanced understanding of how genes, the environment, and several unknown factors converge to result in complex human characteristics—and they've started implementing this approach in classrooms around the country.

It's not only kids who need to learn to honor the complexity of genetics. I strongly believe that progressive parents need to do the same. In the oversimplified view that most of us learned in school, in animals with XY sex determination, the sperm determines the offspring's sex. If it has a Y chromosome, the fertilized egg has an XY genotype and is male in phenotype. If it has an X, the fertilized egg will have an XX genotype and be female in phenotype. In this school of thought, the offspring's sex is thought to be determined at fertilization, meaning it's written in stone in their DNA. But that's not how it works.

It's not merely sex chromosomes that differentiate sex. In 1990, scientists discovered the SRY gene, so named for the sex-determining region at the tip of the short arm of the human Y chromosome. Over thirty years ago, scientists figured that the SRY gene was entirely responsible for male development once it's activated a few weeks after conception and starts making its protein. But that's not even quite how it works.

Each of a human's 23 pairs of chromosomes contains hundreds or thousands of genes, and with the fast advancement of DNA sequencing, scientists have realized that there's a lot more we don't know about our genes than we do know. In just the last couple of decades, we've learned that a slew of genes that aren't even on the sex chromosomes also play major roles in sex differentiation. As science increasingly illuminates how complex sex is, variability rather than bimodality comes to light.

How we think about the genome is evolving, and that means our thinking about not only gender and sex but kids' well-being has to evolve, too.

Though the Mendelian pattern of inheritance, also called the single-gene pattern, is among the most commonly known forms of inheritance, it's actually the most basic and is the exception among organisms, not the rule. Yes, a few human traits are largely controlled by a single gene, like whether you can roll your tongue or whether your earlobes are attached to your neck or freely flopping. But even so-called single-gene traits are more complicated than we've been led to believe, and there are far more traits that are the result of complex interactions of multiple genes with external determinants. **As I've navigated the discourse around not only sex but behavior, disease, and more, I've realized that parents need a refreshed understanding of the inconceivable complexity of the relationship between genotype and phenotype, from athleticism to propensity for**

migraines and any other biological trait under the sun. As parents, we pay attention to phenotype even if we don't think about it that way. Our children's traits, like temperament, height, susceptibility to viruses, eating habits, and others influence everything from academic and athletic attainment to behavioral issues to diseases and conditions they may experience throughout life.

All of the DNA in any cell or living thing is known as a genome, which is often compared to the blueprint for an organism. In humans, the genome is about three billion characters, also known as nucleotides or base pairs, long.

Cells in a human body typically contain a nucleus that houses 23 pairs of chromosomes with one of each pair from each parent, for a total of 46. Each chromosome is made of super-long sequences of four molecular "letters"—adenine (A), cytosine (C), guanine (G), and thymine (T). A DNA molecule is made of two strands of paired nucleotides twisted into the familiar double helix ladder. Based on their complementary molecular structure, A always pairs with T, and C always pairs with G. Each base pair is held together by chemical bonds.

When a cell is building a specific protein, each of which has a specific job in the larger project of building an organism and maintaining its functions, the first step is for a piece of the very long double helix to unzip its structure. Then, an enzyme called *RNA polymerase* in the nucleus of a cell binds to a gene, which is like a paragraph or page of that blueprint. The enzyme moves along the gene and creates a new chain of nucleotides called *mRNA* which is basically a template to build a particular protein.

When the mRNA template is ready, it detaches from the DNA, exits the nucleus, and makes its way to a piece of machinery called the *ribosome* in the cell. The ribosome reads the mRNA in sets of three nucleotides called *codons*. The different codons code for twenty different *amino acids*, which are the building blocks of all of the proteins in living things. The ribosome moves along the mRNA and puts together the corresponding blocks and detaches when it's finished.

Think of it as everyone having blueprints to build a cookie-cutter house, but there are many slight differences in each, like the brand and shades of paint, the size and types of nails in the front porch, the features in the kitchen and bathrooms, the flooring material, the roof, and the foundation. There are thought to be around 20,000 to 25,000 genes. You get two copies of each, one from each biological parent. Every individual's genome is over 99.9% identical to any other human. That 0.1% difference between any two individuals, or about one out of every thousand base pairs, is scattered throughout our vast genomes. This genomic variation is a big part of what makes us unique.

Unlike a widow's peak, the vast majority of phenotypic traits are complex or *polygenic*, which means that variations in multiple genes interact with a web of environmental factors and manifest as, say, a powerful singing voice, a way with words, addiction, social anxiety, or cellulite. Most diseases, including diabetes, heart disease, and many cancers, are similarly complex. Someone's phenotype is basically everything observable about a person. My current phenotype includes a pointy chin, a (so-called) women's US 9.5 shoe size, stretch marks on my abdomen, a need to urinate frequently, a love of music videos and books, anxiety, astigmatism, allergies, and a hankering to dismantle the patriarchy.

Each gene paragraph is made of sentences that cells can cut, copy, and paste in a multitude of configurations to build molecules that do a multitude of things. The Human Genome Project published the first almost-full human genome sequence in 2003. Since then, sequencing technologies have become better and faster, leading to mountains of genetic data. Most of that data has not been tapped. It's as if we have lots and lots of copies of human blueprints, but the majority of it is still only as good as gibberish to us—an inconceivably immense set of sequences of As, Ts, Cs, and Gs. Together, I imagine all of the vast amounts of genomic data as an unimaginably massive library. We've read only a fraction of what it contains and understand only a sliver of what we've read. Often, those slivers of understanding are useful, even lifesaving. But sometimes, those slivers of understanding can enable exploitation. The future holds immense potential for both.

The proportion of influence that a child's genotype has over their phenotype has been a matter of contention in recent years, with a power struggle between scientific narratives playing out. Genetic biomechanical factors within the body impact our well-being, but the answer to how much of an impact they have often depends on which expert you consult. It's a twenty-first-century version of the nature versus nurture debate. I think of it as the extent to which a blueprint influences how a house holds up throughout its existence. Yes, a blueprint will affect the outcomes over the course of a lifetime, but so will factors like the weather, care, and neglect.

When it comes to kids' well-being, the struggle between scientific narratives is fundamentally about justice. If a child's outcomes, from behavior to disease, are primarily the product of innate genomic variation, then systems don't have to change. There's little to be done. If differences in outcomes are largely a product of privilege or inequity—or care or neglect in the blueprint–house analogy—then we can *do something* to ensure that all children get the best chances to thrive.

When it comes to sexual development specifically, scientists are only now putting together how the genome influences phenotype. The construct of 3G sex can't capture the complexity. Embryos all develop in the same way for the first few weeks, developing the same generic tissue that eventually matures into genitals and gonads. Ovaries and testes come from that early tissue, and so do penises and clitorises. The tissue that is separated and layered behind the labia instead wraps and closes around the urethra to form the penile shaft in people considered to be males. But as Cary Gabriel Costello, a professor at the University of Wisconsin-Milwaukee, where he leads the LGBT studies program, writes in his blog, "The Western medical establishment is deeply invested in the ideology of sexual dyadism: the idea that there are two very different sexes with two very different sets of genitalia." He explains that "the language we use" and the typical diagrams that "illustrate genitalia hide the similarities between everyone's genitals." The tissues that form the tip of the penis or the clitoris, which Costello and some other scholars call the "phalloclitoris," tend to be misrepresented in typical illustrations. In "the female drawing, it's presented as a tiny clitoral dot, with the label pointing at a spot the size of a small pea. In the male drawing, it's presented as a huge penis" that extends "beyond the testes, apparently 8 inches or more in length even in its flaccid state." He writes that "to put it plainly, the 'normal penis' in" typical medical drawings "is porn-star sized rather than average, and massive in comparison to the petite 'normal clitoris.'"

Rather than a binary, genitals exist on a spectrum. Awareness of people who are intersex, or who have reproductive or sexual anatomy that doesn't conform to typical female or male categories, has gone up, mainly due to increased visibility of the movement focused on ending unnecessary and harmful surgical "normalization" of so-called ambiguous genitalia in babies. As intersex activists have pointed out, no child's genitalia is ambiguous without comparison to a constructed standard. It is simply genitalia. Moreover, many people who are considered intersex have pretty typical genitalia that doesn't look unusual at all. Labia can be fused in a way that looks like a scrotum. A scrotum can be configured in a way that looks like labia. In some individuals, instead of a so-called normal vagina, there is a shallow vagina or smooth patch of lubricating skin. There have been recorded cases of people with both sperm and eggs. Some people with

XX chromosomes have an SRY gene translocated onto an X chromosome and develop typical male genitalia. Some people have XXY, or just one X and no second sex chromosome. Some people have some cells with XX and some with XY. Advances in DNA sequencing and cell biology are revealing that many individuals, including those who can reproduce sexually, are a mosaic of cells with sex variations. All of these truths and more have been stifled and pathologized.

Humans with power decide, by measuring the size of a penis or a clitoris or looking at the relative location of a urethra and other anatomy, whether genitals fall into arbitrary parameters. Around 1 in 1500 to 1 in 2000 infants are flagged at birth as having atypical external genitalia. Yet others are born with more subtle anatomical variations.

Even *sex chromosomes* are a human-made concept. The Y chromosome was thought to be *the* chromosome that makes males male, initially because it looked smaller under a micro-scope in males. We call it *Y* because it resembles a Y when compared to all of the other chromosomes that look more like *X*s. Next came the idea that SRY is the one trigger. That idea also turned out to be less than accurate. Scientists now know there are genes involved in the formation of gonads, genitals, and myriad other sex-associated traits across the genome, not just the X and Y chromosomes. SRY isn't the single master sex-determining gene that it seemed to be. Instead, it's more of a facilitator gene that triggers the activation of other consequential genes on other chromosomes.

Then there are testosterone and estrogen, the hormones that are deeply culturally entrenched as what makes males and fe-males different. There's a common belief that testosterone it-self activates what we think of as *masculine* traits like aggression, strength, and even logical thinking, while estrogen mediates *feminine* ones like nurturing, softness, and emotion. But studies show that these traits are influenced as much by socialization as by hormone levels and that behavior and environment can also increase or decrease testosterone levels in people of all genders. Sexually dimorphic views of estrogen and testosterone levels have long been skewed by the natural monthly menstrual cycle. Scientists think that individual variation over time is more meaningful in terms of how our bodies and minds respond. Dialing up testosterone in an individual dials up what we think of as masculine traits; this is why hormone therapies can be important interventions. This doesn't mean that an individual with certain traditionally masculine traits necessarily has more testosterone than an individual with traditionally feminine traits. That's not how it works. Here again, that old correlation versus causation question comes up. So many of our traits that *seem* to be mechanistically sexed are not caused by sex at all but by other factors, like socialization, size, diet, recreation, occupation, and so much more.

The fact that humans exist on a sex spectrum matters for everyone, especially our children. Think back to what came to mind when you asked yourself to define male and female. In addition to chromosomes and reproductive traits, you might have thought of any of the following: deeper or higher tone of voice, the size of someone's larynx and surrounding cartilage (also known as the Adam's apple), smaller or larger muscle mass, differences in brain size and structure, estrogen or testosterone, or myriad other characteristics that are traditionally associated with being *male* or *female*. Not only are we still learning about how the genome influences these traits, Brusman points out that researchers have only recently gained an understanding of the epigenome, or chemical markers that determine what genes are expressed or not expressed, and how it affects sex.

The epigenome affects far more than sex. On one of our regular Zoom calls, I ask Alison Bernstein, of the Bernstein lab at the Rutgers University School of Pharmacy, what we know so far about epigenetics and their impact on our children's outcomes. It turns out the research is "not even in its infancy," she tells me. "It's still in the fetal development stage." Scientists are only starting to figure it out, and there's a long way to go.

"There are all sorts of downstream factors: maybe gene A does turn on, but it's somehow not able to activate gene B," Brusman explains. With "all these different phenotypes and traits, people like to think it's like a light switch, like either a gene is on or off," but it's really more "like a dimmer." More often than not, these dimmers are "kind of in between" the on or off positions. And these switches all interact with each other and with the external environment in dynamic ways from birth to death that we still barely understand. If anything, the diversity of sex-determination mechanisms only underscores how much scientists have to learn about why it works in the complex ways it does.

Yet some scientists continue to target traits to find a consistent difference. Consider ongoing research that asks whether there are really reliable differences in the brains of males and females. It's a long-known fact that there's no such thing as male and female brains. This has been confirmed time and again, including by a metasynthesis of over three decades of research published in 2021 in the journal *Neuroscience & Biobehavioral Reviews*. Despite the body of evidence that demolishes the myth of the sexually dimorphic brain, the authors of the article write that many neuroscientists still assume "that larger studies, using higher-resolution imaging and better processing pipelines will uncover the 'real,' or specieswide differences between male and female brain structure and connectivity patterns. However, the present synthesis indicates that such 'real' or universal sex-related differences do not exist."

There are also scientific narratives fighting it out when it comes to so-called girls' and boys' or men's and women's sports.

Personally, I agree with the growing yet still-unpopular stance that sex-segregated sports don't make sense. There's no evidence that trans girls have a performance edge over cis girls of the same age or that trans boys are at an inherent disadvantage on boys' teams. The same goes for adults. The notion that segregating the sexes in sports is done because males are bigger, stronger, and faster than females is based on mythology. Dr. Sheree Bekker, associate editor of the *British Journal of Sports Medicine*, is among experts who staunchly disagree with the narrative that women's sport "exists as a 'protected category' so that women can win."

As she tweeted on March 18, 2022, this "is not the reason why women's sport exists as a category," and "it is not true that no woman will ever win again."

This narrative is "profoundly paternalistic and keeps women small." She explains that it's important for people to be aware that women's sport exists as a category because women competing began to threaten the dominance of men.

Bekker continues to give several examples.

For instance, in 1902 Madge Syers was the first woman to enter a figure skating world championship. At the time, there wasn't a rule against women competing, though it had never happened before. She took 2nd place, and continued beating men at competitions. "By 1903 women were banned from the World Championships," she writes. "Then, in 1905, we have a segregated women's category."

Bekker writes that "the pattern is clear: where women were included (or simply included themselves) it was only when they started threatening men's dominance/entitlement that they were segregated into a separate category." It has never been "about a benevolent (still sexist) aim of supposedly 'giving women a chance to win.' It was about control."

She goes on to explain that there are some real-life examples and research studies that suggest that inclusion is "not only the right thing to do, but it also makes us all better."

**Many parents wonder what the right reaction would be
if their kid is gender-nonconforming or trans.** But there's
a lot that comes ahead of that question. There is plenty that we
can do as parents who care about social justice and believe in
science no matter our own child's gender identity or sexuality.

Signal safety and support in your own backyard. Continue to interrogate your worldviews. Actively don a fresh lens.
No matter how much we identify with believing in science and
social justice, we can't rest on progressive identity laurels.

With some progressive parents, it's "a 'not in my backyard'
kind of thing," Summers tells me. "When LGBTQ rights are
an abstraction, it's easy to be supportive of it." The pediatrician
and father, who works in the northern suburbs of Boston—"a
very sort of progressive kind of community, if you will"—says
children have confided in him that while their parents "are progressive on paper, 'I don't feel like I can share this part of myself
with them.'" In those cases, he tries to talk about how "hopefully, it will get better." For many families, contending with a
child's gender identity and sexuality "can be a struggle, but over
time, things improve."

If you're not open about gender and progressive values in
your own backyard and fail to push back against binarism in
your family, friend group, PTO, school district, and other spaces
where you have influence, then your kids may not end up trusting you with who they are. Recent generations have been far
more comfortable with cutting out problematic biological family
members than previous generations. For children who feel unsafe being out to their families, Summers says, "It may be that, as
time goes by, the role that families typically fill for people may
not be your biological family. Hopefully, that's not going to be
the case." But sometimes it is the case, and he tells patients that
"chosen family" is "one way that you can think about how you
get the support and community that you need if it's not available in your home."

It's about us as progressive parents doing "super basic things," says Muldrow. Depending on your comfort level in your community, it "can be really powerful" to signal that you're "a safe adult, not just for your kids, but for their friends." It can be as simple as "wearing a *Protect Trans Kids* T-shirt" or "having a bumper sticker on your car so that when you pull up to the school, kids know that's a safe person, and that's a person who can see me."

I ask Muldrow about what she would say to those who think that things like bumper stickers and T-shirts are performative. "I feel like people can be critical of those things, but I think they're necessary signals" that are "really powerful." She also points out that not everyone has the same bandwidth and that our actions add up no matter how small. "We can't have a movement that is ableist. We can't have a movement that says, 'Wait, if you can't show up at the march, then you're not one of us,'" she says. "We have to have a movement that's as diverse as we are. We have to have access points to this movement that are as diverse as we are."

C. P., a dear friend of mine who raised a trans kid in Madison, says that, if it's possible, parents providing "a safe place for" their child's friends to go "if their bio family is abusive or otherwise unsupportive" can be a lifesaver. Part of signaling safety is gender-neutral language.

None of this means erasing women and girls—a common argument that crumbles under scrutiny. Pushing back against binarism doesn't mean that sex, gender, and sexuality aren't real. They are tangible, integral parts of who we are at our core and continue to hold value when applied thoughtfully and with accuracy. When you're referring to an individual and you know their pronouns, use their pronouns. So yes, if you are lactating and are a woman and mom, then people should refer to you as a *lactating woman and mom*. If your child menstruates and is a girl, refer to her as a *girl with a period*. If your child is a boy and menstruates, refer to him as a *boy with a period*. If your child is gender-nonconforming, refer to them by whatever their pronouns are. But if you're referring to people in general, be inclusive. Think *everyone* instead of *ladies and gentlemen*, *kids* instead of *boys and girls*, or *firefighters* instead of *firemen*. It might feel weird. It definitely felt weird to me circa 2018 when I was writing about human-health research for a client that was transitioning to gender-neutral language. It wasn't long before using phrases like *children and adults who menstruate* or *women, girls, and other people who menstruate* instead of *women and girls* when talking about people who get their period began to feel like second nature. It wasn't much longer before media references to only *women's* right to choose became troubling.

As someone who studies disparities in reproductive health, Green tells me, "the researcher I am now, I wasn't that researcher a decade ago, five years ago." At first, she found it hard to use gender-neutral language for birthing people because her work "centers Black women, and Black women are so often marginalized in this discourse." But eventually, "I was willing to examine my own biases" and "my wish for accuracy and empathy won over any desire" to stick to strictly binary language about reproduction.

In raising our own kids with gender-neutral language, "I keep worrying about doing it badly," Green says. "My spouse is like, 'Okay, they're kind of young.'" She recalls telling him that "you're not too young to be exposed to these really toxic ideas about gender. You're socialized into gender from birth."

I get the feeling Green is doing it the opposite of badly. She wants her kids to know that she doesn't have a problem questioning her assumptions. It's "okay to be wrong. Normalize being wrong for your kids. Normalize being wrong and not being ashamed of that," she says.

Part of positioning ourselves as parents who carry ourselves through the world based on as much of the truth as we can access is knowing the truth about how gender and sexuality develop. There is a misconception that transness is new. It's not. There have always been trans people.

There has been a lot of sciencey-sounding rhetoric that aims to convince parents and politicians that talking to children about gender and sexuality will "turn them" trans or gay, which is bigoted propaganda. Consider the myth of so-called rapid onset gender dysphoria (ROGD), which purportedly occurs as a matter of social contagion. ROGD "is a politicized pseudo-diagnostic category," writes Florence Ashley, a transfeminine jurist, bioethicist, and doctoral candidate at the University of Toronto, in a 2020 commentary in *The Sociological Review Monographs*. "Introduced in 2016, the term reflects a deliberate attempt to weaponize scientific-sounding language to dismiss mounting empirical evidence of the benefits of transition for youth."

Trust credible medical professionals and progressive school districts. "There's a huge campaign right now that's all about making us distrust public schools and distrust educators" and "distrust medical professionals," says Muldrow. Trust isn't a given, especially in health care, but it makes sense to trust that gender-affirming clinicians and educators "know what is developmentally appropriate."

"For years now, for all of my adolescent visits, I ask about gender and sexual identity as a matter of routine. And I front-load that conversation with a little disclaimer," says Summers. "These are questions that I ask everybody, please don't take any question personally. None of this is based on anything about you specifically. These are questions I literally ask every single person," he assures patients. "I have yet to have a single teenage patient of mine blink at those questions."

In America, generation after generation, we've been talking to kids since infancy about gender and sexuality, and the way we've been doing it has been riddled with inaccuracies and ideology. For too many children, those inaccuracies have been constraints. "When we say pronouns save lives, or one trusted adult makes a difference, we aren't talking in theoretical terms," says Abigail Swetz, a former middle-school teacher, foster mom, advocate, poet, and former Wisconsin Department of Public Instruction communications director. To parents and other adults who aren't sure if words and actions matter, "there are children still alive and learning in a classroom" in school districts like ours "because a teacher used 'they/them'" to describe a student "or wore a rainbow ribbon on a lanyard or insisted on creating a safe space." She makes herself totally clear: "These aren't hypotheticals. These are real, living children. And there are other kids who are not. Because they are dead." Those who are fighting for trans rights aren't trying to turn kids trans. They're trying to turn kids into adults.

Vote against bigoted legislation. Bills targeting trans and gender-nonconforming youth, including those that seek to restrict gender-affirming care, access to bathrooms, and participation in sports, have been proliferating in the US. For too many families, these attacks have been a nightmare. In some areas, the law makes every citizen a mandatory reporter of doctors, educators, and parents. This means someone's own neighbor or community member could be required by law to turn families in for supporting their children's identities. Children shouldn't have to worry about, let alone endure, family separation or their parents getting arrested for affirming who they are.

The Trans Formations Project, a nonprofit organization dedicated to tracking and educating about the antitrans legislative crisis sweeping the country, provides a tool that helps people "find and track hateful and helpful legislation proposals that impact the health and safety of vulnerable youth and their families" locally, and to find and hold state-level representatives accountable. It also provides much-needed updates about legislative wins for trans rights. Find the Project at www.transformationsproject.org.

The Facebook group Transgender Parenting is an educational group led by the expertise of trans and nonbinary adults that helps support trans children by providing correct education to caregivers and correcting harmful misinformation. Please agree to and abide by group rules upon joining: https://www.facebook.com/groups/transgenderparenting/.

Contribute to organizations that support local trans folks, like those that can help secure housing, bail, protection, and other dire needs.

Finally, we arrive at what to do if your kid is trans, nonbinary, gender-nonconforming, or queer.

Without a doubt, the best you can do for a trans or gendernonconforming child is to follow their lead, support them, validate their experiences, seek out affirming health-care providers for them, educate yourself, and provide resources. As former professional basketball player Dwayne Wade said publicly to his trans daughter when she legally changed her name to Zaya, "as your father, my job isn't to create a version of myself or direct your future, my role is to be a facilitator to your hopes, your wishes, and your dreams." It's understandable to feel anxiety or even grief over an idealized future someone imagined for their child. It's ideal to work out those feelings with a therapist and not burden the child with them. Parents may also need to protect children from people who are unwilling to support them, including other adults in the family.

Ask your child what they need and how you can help. Sometimes, it can start with helping kids "find the words they need to describe themselves in a place that is largely supportive," C. P. tells me. Whatever they decide, respect their choices. "Acknowledge whatever ignorance you have," she says. Parents "don't have to understand" their kid's journey to support them. They "just need to be there" to let the child know "that they are loved no matter what."

The process of gender-affirming care is far less drastic than widely believed. Major medical organizations, including the American Academy of Pediatrics, the American Medical Association, and the American Endocrine Association, agree that this care is evidence-based, and starkly reduces suicidality, depression, and self-harming behavior. Ideally, decisions about whether to seek gender-affirming care and what that care entails are made between a provider, a patient, and their parents or guardians. These decisions depend on the individual's situation and needs. Gender-affirming care can include support with social transition. Some youth may eventually receive treatments to temporarily stall puberty, which typically begin once the individual has already started puberty. Some may choose gender-affirming hormone replacement therapy, which can happen at sixteen or seventeen with parental consent, sometimes younger. Top surgery, or the surgical removal of breast tissue, may be an option for transmasculine youth as young as sixteen with parental consent. Genital surgery, sometimes known as sex reassignment surgery, isn't recommended for minors.

What science shows without question is that affirmation of gender and sexuality saves lives and gives children the opportunity and space to thrive. Remember that seeking accepting health-care providers doesn't mean pushing children to medically transition. The idea "that we're rushing kids to these medical treatments that are irreversible" and that "we're rushing kids to surgery" is "absolutely fallacious," says Summers. Anyone who thinks so "clearly knows nothing about this system," he says with the tone of a man who has heard it too many times.

The bottom line is we know now that rocks can't sexually reproduce, and that many of Linneaus's conjectures about biological categorization have proven almost comically wrong. The more we learn, the more biology reveals itself to be far more prismatic than it seems. Children continue to learn outdated notions of biological hierarchy, while systems continue to perpetuate it. Not only do identities defy static categorization, but so do human bodies.

Sex and gender are only the beginning when it comes to

the harms of biological essentialism on children, and that old question about the influence of genotype on phenotype. When it comes to kids' well-being, there's another pseudoscientific method of categorization that seems totally biologically sound and that Linnaeus also helped originate: race, and its modern forms, ethnicity and ancestry.

4

beginning to navigate race,
ethnicity, and ancestry

Madison takes pride in its progressive values, and for four years after arriving in 1987, it seemed downright idyllic to me and my playmates. The twenty-acre University Houses apartment community, along with the neighboring Eagle Heights, will forever be the perfect pocket of the world to the children who have lived there. Reality would soon come for us, but not then. Back then, it seemed entirely ordinary to freely roam the wooded area that surrounded our buildings and the courtyards between them with my multicultural pack of friends. Each summer, we became the masters of this domain, getting around on foot, bikes (mine was called Pink Lightning), roller skates, or Radio Flyer wagon. Wherever we wandered, we were wards of the adults in closest proximity, but we barely noticed their eyes peering at us through curtains. During the school year, friends would pop into our apartment before school to catch an episode of *The Jetsons* and imagine a future with flying cars and friendly robots. Our place was also a popular hangout because it was the only place on the block with a Nintendo Entertainment System, which my *athai* (father's sister) and *mama* (my uncle) surprised me with on one of their regular visits from Illinois. My *amichi* (maternal grandmother) came to Madison from India and stayed with us for much of 1989 when my sister was an infant, and she found these gatherings amusing.

At Shorewood Hills, the near west-side Madison elementary school nicknamed the Little United Nations because of its international student population, where many of my classmates were the kids of UW faculty and staff, we went by name and country or countries of ancestry. There were a few white classmates, and they were also grilled about their European backgrounds, in an unusual reversal of the *Where are you really from?* line of questioning that non-white Americans are accustomed to. The only ones we counted as really from America were Native Americans. (I don't recall how we referred to those whose ancestry was unknown. Looking back, I get the feeling that, at the time even our relatively progressive little school participated in the erasure of the experiences of Black Americans with enslaved ancestors.) I was Kavin "from" India (despite being born at Georgetown University Hospital in Washington, DC), along with Jala, Raju, and others from India. There was Dominic from Portugal, Sarah and Yvette from Mexico, Laura and Joe from the Central African Republic, and Lea from Denmark. In the unit next door to ours, with a small pantry connecting the two apartments, lived my best friend, Hrafnhildur (Hilda) from Iceland, her brother Víkingur, and eventually their baby siblings Marinella and Jón Ágúst. Frequent visitors to our neighborhood from other parts of Madison included my other best friend Nirthika (Nirmi) from Sri Lanka and our dear friend Megha from India, among many others. Our pack of young ears easily grasped all of our neighbors' accents. At dusk, the grown-ups shattered our fun, shouting us in for dinner. "Right now! Don't make me count! I'm counting… Uno! Dos!"

We attended school in a melting pot. Back when my city's culinary scene consisted largely of European-American fare, the lunch tables at Shorewood Hills cafeteria brimmed with lovingly packed flavors that most Madisonians had never experienced. In kindergarten, we learned that we were the high-school graduating Class of 2000. The grown-ups thought that this was quite exciting. We were the generation of the future, they told us. We could be anything we wanted to be and do anything we put our minds to. (Surely, one of us would invent flying cars.)

High school seemed so far away that it felt silly to make a big deal about graduating from it, but the staff at Shorewood relished their unique opportunity. An article from 1991 about a "new crop of teachers putting multicultural education into practice" features my third-grade teacher, Ms. Hartmann, who explains that kids have to feel good about themselves to succeed, and part of that is learning about their culture. My childhood classmate Yani (from Malaysia), found the yellowed clipping in 2020. In the photo accompanying the piece, my classmates and I surround a determined young Hartmann. We're disheveled and wiggly from our day of learning, hardly aware that anything unusual is underway. "If in school all the kids learn about is white culture," Hartmann is quoted as saying, "how can they be proud about who they are?"

Looking back on the old page, a bittersweet lump formed in my throat. At one of the most harrowing points in the COVID-19 lockdown, the then thirtysomethings in the photo were gathered in a Facebook thread to reflect on that moment captured in the clipping. One of my classmates shared that she's thankful because our neighborhood and school "gave us a base point for what should be considered normal in this racist country and what we could aspire to be." It's a sliver of our lives that we protect in our hearts, a time that will never shatter. "I feel so blessed to have had time together before the world showed its harshness," another of my old buddies said. "This was a truly special time and place where kids really found commonality and pride in our uniqueness." We had no idea how good we had it, in far more ways than one.

I think of Madison, with its majestic granite state capitol dome rising from the isthmus between the sparkling waters of Lakes Mendota and Monona, as my home. The sun is brilliant this June 14, 2020. My family and I haven't ventured downtown from our place on the southwest side since before the first COVID-19 lockdown in March, and it feels strange yet comforting to be here. I soak up the sun, bottling its warmth to uncork in the winter when our city freezes over, and intrepid ice fishers dot the frozen lakes. I'm stressed over this brand-new pandemic, which ripped the floor out from under us, more violently for some than others, and reeling, yet hopeful, over the Black Lives Matter movement that tenacious activists invigorated following the murder of George Floyd. I'm also healing from the years-long, grueling reconfiguration of myself.

We're downtown with our children to participate in the filming of a campaign video for Nada Elmikashfi, a climate activist who was then running for the state senate, and who currently serves as chief of staff to Wisconsin State Representative Francesca Hong. Their father and I corral our fidgety nine- and seven-year-olds. We approach Nada and her crew on the front steps of the capitol, the bronze *Wisconsin* statue gleaming brightly atop the granite dome, her right hand extended as if to usher progress. At ground level stands another statue, the seven-foot bronze sculpture of a woman with her right arm outstretched and left arm clutching an American flag, her pedestal bearing the state motto, Forward. She's stood on the capitol grounds since 1895 (with a replica standing in since the 1990s), embodying the motto year in and year out. Protesters would tear down the statue, known lovingly as Lady Forward, days later.

Elmikashfi's unapologetic stances on social and environmental justice are particularly compelling to me not only because of how much she cares about the kids in our community but because of how worried she is about the children she hopes to have someday. She doesn't mince words, explaining that she fears having to bury her Black children before they bury her. We both know what it's like to grow up in a city that we love all while coming to terms with what she calls "a deeply hurtful, systemic inequity," one that starts hitting in early childhood.

Spending time in and around the capitol building is among my first memories and among my own kids' earliest recollections, too. Like so many other children who have toured the capitol building with their parents or on school field trips from all over the state, as I peered into the chambers of the Wisconsin legislature, it was clear to me that important people do important things here. When protesters toppled Lady Forward on June 23, 2020, some progressive Madisonians, parents like myself among them, were baffled. Why target a statue that stands for progress? I also initially felt dismayed.

"Lady Forward is the symbolic gatekeeper of an almost all-white capitol that legislates in racism," tweeted Elmikashfi. I felt my stomach drop as I read her words. "Knocking it down made so many allies uncomfortable tonight[.]" I was uncomfortable, too. "That is effective protest," she concluded. Her new rallying cry, *Fuck your statues*, seeded controversy on local social media as towns across America grappled with their own problematic statues.

Though Elmikashfi's unvarnished support of the protesters may feel gratuitously militant, contending with any resulting discomfort is a necessary "sacrifice" that progressive parents need to make, says Francesca Hong, parent, chef, community organizer, and representative of the 76th district of the Wisconsin State Assembly. The capitol building is among Madison's most prized icons, but to some, it represents an untenable status quo.

I'm among the folks who have eventually come around to understand Elmikashfi's perspective. "Quite a few" people have reached out to Elmikashfi to say that, while her view on statues once rubbed them the wrong way, it began to make sense on some level. The tearing down of Lady Forward was an outcry from the city's soul: *What we've been doing since 1895 isn't moving us all forward.* A statue bearing the motto Forward in front of the state capitol building all while age-old inequity is alive and well, harming children across Wisconsin, feels like a scam. We haven't been upholding the motto's ideal when swathes of babies continue to be left behind, generation after generation. Grappling with this stark reality is necessary to begin to set an example for our own kids.

When I was in fourth grade, my father left the university, and we moved to a less diverse part of the city. I started attending a far more homogenous elementary school. Most of the students were white (middle school and high school eventually allowed me to mingle with non-European-American classmates again). On my first day of fourth grade at the new school, my mom packed chicken and rice in my lunchbox. "Ewww" came the declaration from the other end of the long lunch table. "What's that smell?" Other children followed suit, pinching their noses in disgust. My heart jumped into my throat. Similarly, though it had never bothered me before, I soon became embarrassed by my dad's accent. I was nine when I first began to feel the effects of racism and xenophobia, protected in large part until then by that perfect pocket of the world I lived in starting at age five. When I reminisce with other adults who, in their own childhoods, lived at Eagle Heights or the University Houses and attended Shorewood Hills over the years, our own Little United Nations, I feel a sense of gratitude for the priceless experience and a twinge of sadness for the innocence we lost.

After saying our goodbyes to Elmikashfi and their crew, we head to Madison's iconic State Street for a stroll with the kids. I've walked this pedestrian zone, which extends west from the capitol and joins the UW campus at Library Mall countless times before, as a child taking three tiny steps to my dad's long stride, in high school after a bus ride with friends, and as a student at the university stopping for a burrito on the way to class. As we walk, State Street is unrecognizable following the fresh upheaval of the summer of 2020. Murals painted on the boarded-up storefronts have transformed the city's wounds into art. *We Are Black Girl Magic* declares one. A wide-eyed Martin Luther King Jr. in a green nightshirt, an American flag blanket pulled up to his chin, speaks via speech bubble to all who pass: *I had a nightmare.* Weary Madison residents, many with their solemn children, stroll and ponder the paintings and names of George Floyd, Breonna Taylor, Madison's own Tony Robinson, and too many others that cops have murdered. With no shows to publicize during the COVID lockdown, the marquee of the historic Orpheum Theater reads *Black Lives Matter.*

In February of 2017, the feeding-your-kids news cycle was flooded with reports of a new study in the *Journal of Pediatrics* that claimed that Black infants had over twice the deaths of white babies attributable to lack of "optimal" breastfeeding. The study concluded that suboptimal breastfeeding was associated with significant differences in childhood diseases, including a type of leukemia, ear infections, gastrointestinal infection, lower respiratory tract infections, and SIDS. Headlines like one declaring that "Alarming disparities in health outcomes could be prevented by breastfeeding" made the rounds, reinforcing the Breast Is Best mantra with a racial-justice framing.

But this narrative about the study that the death of Black babies is directly attributable to suboptimal breastfeeding has "a transparent, fatal flaw," pediatrician Daniel Summers told me in 2017. As we've learned, the benefits associated with breastfeeding are only *associated with* and not predominantly *caused by* breastfeeding. Rather than rely on real-life health outcomes, the study used computerized simulations to evaluate two hypothetical cohorts of US women and their hypothetical infants.

While there's no doubt that barriers to breastfeeding should be dismantled, the conclusions are based on a fundamentally faulty assumption: that observed associations between breastfeeding and well-being are causal.

"[B]y making the leap from association/correlation to causation across too wide an array of outcomes, the authors have made an error that utterly undermines the conclusions," Summers told me. "It rests on a very shaky assumption, and its resulting conclusions are unsound."

Again, it's crucial to support breastfeeding for anyone who wants to do so. What's unsettling is that it's not the lack of optimal breastfeeding that's disproportionately killing and sickening babies and children of certain races. It's racism.

In the summer of 2019, Jeanette Kowalik, PhD, MPH, then Milwaukee's health commissioner, was in the weeds of the fight for the city to declare racism a public-health crisis. In Milwaukee and practically all other major American cities, where someone lives has a lot to do with race. Redlining, a federally sanctioned practice that started in the 1930s, highlighted the areas where Black and other non-white people would live. Native-American children have also often lived in segregated tribal areas as a result of government-sanctioned theft of land, discrimination, and economic and environmental neglect that is still alive and well today. In municipalities all over the US, forms of historical segregation and discrimination including redlining still influence how resources, like access to high-quality health care, are allocated and how exposure to hazards, like lead, is distributed. Milwaukee, which is still one of the most segregated metropolitan areas in the United States, has one of the highest Black mortality rates in the nation. Disparities in health and achievement are "basically the direct result of the redlining maps," Kowalik tells me over the phone in June of 2021. All of this was by design, and the results are plain to see. Maps of neighborhood health throughout the US show that the highest concentrations of lead poisoning, higher rates of asthma, diabetes, obesity, COVID-19 deaths, and shorter lifespan align distinctly with age-old segregation. The relationship between systemic racism and these poor health outcomes is most certainly causal.

Though poverty affects people of all races, it doesn't affect everyone in the same way. Black, Hispanic, Indigenous, and other specific groups of marginalized non-white people are more likely than white people with comparable incomes to live in neighborhoods with concentrated disadvantages and harms and limited opportunities like employment options and good schools.

Not all forms of geographic injustice are obvious, but some forms of residential inequity are plain to see. Consider tree equity. Health-related factors, like air quality and surface temperature have been directly linked to the number and size of trees in a neighborhood. Areas with higher tree coverage have better air quality and lower summer surface temperatures. Generally, there are fewer trees in historically segregated neighborhoods. Trees or their absence are a visible predictor of housing inequity.

Before she became health commissioner, Kowalik was a single mother living in predominantly Black neighborhoods, working her way through her education at the University of Wisconsin-Milwaukee, eventually earning her doctorate in health sciences. Like so many Black people in the city, she almost got caught in "the trap of the system," she tells me on a call while I was reporting for a magazine story in 2021. When she was pregnant with her son born in 1998, she struggled to access basic needs including high-quality health care.

In 2019, as Wisconsin's precious short summer warmed up, Kowalik and her colleagues drafted a resolution calling the city's stark racial disparities a "public health crisis." The word *crisis* was chosen deliberately to signal that the widespread harms of racism threaten the long-term health of a large number of people: it is far more dire and widespread than a public health *issue* and far more prolonged than an *emergency*. Convincing the Milwaukee City Council to agree wasn't easy, Kowalik says. Some council members objected, and she and her non-white colleagues had to share their personal experiences to persuade them. As a Black woman born and raised in Milwaukee, it was "demoralizing" to try to change other people's minds. Nobody should have to bare their trauma as an exercise in persuasion. Yet Kowalik and her colleagues ultimately succeeded. Milwaukee adopted the resolution, becoming the first city in the nation to declare racism a health crisis in July 2019. As the 2020 racial reckoning gained momentum, hundreds of jurisdictions did the same.

Racism is far more than redlining and more than what's obvious to the senses. It harms children in dynamic, complex ways no matter their class, location, or living situation. Just like the constructs of the sex and gender binary, the problem with the social and scientific construct of race—and its pervasive by-product, racism—comes down to biological essentialism. **Like sex, it's that old notion that humanity can be grouped into natural, hierarchical categories.** As it is with "biological sex," when it comes to kids' well-being, the notion that race is a biological thing is an insidious lie.

"The truth that it is perfectly possible for prominent scientists to be racist, to murder, to abuse both people and knowledge doesn't sit easily with the way we like to think about scientific research," writes British journalist and author Angela Saini in her acclaimed 2019 book, *Superior: The Return of Race Science.* "We imagine that it's above politics, that it's a noble, rational, and objective endeavor, untainted by feelings or prejudice." This book changed my life, catalyzing the slow breaking of my unwavering trust in science, like the gradual propagation of cracks across tempered glass.

In *Superior*, Saini paints a chilling picture of how all of the atrocities of racism are rooted in one basic myth: that race is bi-

ologically real, residing in people's bones and blood. She high-
lights that tenacious generations of antiracists have been fighting
this lie for ages.

Kids' and parents' lives are in the balance. Those born
to parents who are Black, Hispanic, or Indigenous are significantly more likely to die than white people's babies. (Note that
this broad statement can hardly capture the varying disparities
and unique issues facing children of different groups.) There
are also disparities in the rate of death from pregnancy-related
causes: Black birthing people are around three times as likely
to die as their white counterparts. Racism has harmed Black
women's health since slavery, and Black women have been advocating for autonomy, dignity, and rights in reproductive health
for as long. It is their long-standing labor that forced acknowl-
edgment of the role of racism as a structural determinant of
health.

Parents and children often face racism at the hands of clinicians. Study after study continues to confirm that, in the US,
white patients tend to receive preferential treatment from doctors, nurses, and other providers. Minority patients, especially
Black people, tend to receive subpar care and treatment options
and are often blamed for their own ailments. Black babies and
birthing people fare better when they have Black providers.

Rachel Hardeman, PhD, MPH, a reproductive-health equity
researcher at the University of Minnesota, whose research eluci-
dates the role of racism on health for birthing people and their
babies, warns against making the wrong assumption about these
stark racial gaps. In emails in 2022, she says that a "critical point
missing from these conversations far too often is that it is **racism**,
not **race** [Hardeman's emphasis] that puts Black birthing people
at greater risk for adverse birth outcomes." Her stance echoes
the views of several researchers, clinicians, and other activists.
There is nothing encoded in our DNA, nothing in the fibers
of our muscles, the marrow of our bones, that makes us this or

that race. When people say that race is a social construct, they don't mean that race "isn't real." Rather, they mean that those in power have engaged in an ongoing political process that has racialized all non-white humans. They mean that the progenitors of the concept held so much power that their pseudoscientific declaration permeated humanity. Like biological sex, once the idea of biological race took hold, all of the most powerful institutions joined forces to fabricate a racial hierarchy, ultimately rendering race as real as other social constructs that shape our reality, like money or national borders. Believing that race is biological doesn't automatically make someone "a racist." We've all been conditioned to assume that race is in our blood. Though race is a biological fiction, its power is undeniable.

Progress is ongoing, but unacceptably slow. Medical students and biomedical researchers are still taught that someone's race is itself causing negative health outcomes, and this carries over into the care they provide as doctors. Even though the idea of race is so ingrained, most people, including scientists, struggle to define it.

Racial essentialism can lead people to perceive those of other races as less worthy of affection and assistance. Psychology literature shows that essentialist thinking correlates with greater dehumanization and increased racial prejudice. In a study of college students, those who were primed to perceive race as a social construct rather than a genetic reality were shown to be more distressed by social inequity. Participants primed to view race as a biological construct were more likely to be okay with inequity. "In the face of devastating educational, economic, housing, and health inequities in communities of color, genetic conceptions of race are direct threats to justice," writes Jennifer Tsai, an emergency-medicine physician, BLM activist, and sometimes street medic, in a 2022 article in the *American Medical Association Journal of Ethics*.

The modern idea of race appeared hundreds of years ago. In

the eighteenth century, influential European intellectuals, including Linnaeus, started to categorize races systematically by skin color and other characteristics. Known as one of the greatest thinkers of all time, German philosopher Immanuel Kant, who was also instrumental in the invention of race, subdivided the newly defined Homo sapiens into four groups: "white" Europeans, "yellow" Asians, "red" Native Americans, and "black" Africans. Kant suggested that the environments that influenced skin color also changed the biological essence of these groups, including the "juices" of the body. The latitudes of Africa account "for the origin of the Negro, who is well-suited to his climate," he wrote. "However, because he is so amply supplied by his motherland, he is also lazy, indolent, and dawdling." Kant concluded that Northwestern Europe just happened to produce the ideal human stock, the result of "the perfect mixing of juices."

By the nineteenth century, "those who didn't live like Europeans were thought not yet to have fully realized their potential as human beings," notes Saini. "What Europeans saw as cultural shortcomings in other populations in the early nineteenth century soon became conflated with how they looked."

Ideas about race have evolved since then, growing more detailed, refined, subtle, and, well, science-y, maintaining their stronghold even as their essence remains utter drivel. Categorizing humans by skin color makes about as much scientific sense as categorizing them by the depth of their belly button or the shape of their fingerprints.

Like so many others who believed the pervasive dogma that race and ethnicity are biological, so much of what I thought I knew was not only wrong, it was racist. The world as we know it, a world in which the legacies of whiteness, colonialism, and racism still impact our kids, depends on the collective fallacy that decent, educated, and above all else *rational* people are not racist. As author Ibram X. Kendi often says, "the very heartbeat of racism is denial." It constantly morphs into forms that hardly look like racism at all. It's latent, cloaked by a thin veneer of plausible deniability.

In his 2019 book, *How to Be An Antiracist*, Kendi defines racism as "a marriage of racist policies and racist ideas that produces and normalizes racial inequities." He defines racist policies as "any measure that produces or sustains racial inequity between racial groups." These can be "written and unwritten laws, rules, procedures, processes, regulations, and guidelines that govern people." They take the form of decorum, dominant culture, prejudice, standards, assumptions, access, and exclusion.

If mitigating the harms of racism matters to someone, it's not enough to be *not racist*, they must be actively *antiracist*.

Kendi writes that racist ideas "argue that the inferiorities and superiorities of racial groups explain racial inequities in society." These are the very racist ideas that progressive parents need to dismantle. The challenge is that racist ideas are usually subtle and pernicious. The rhetoric often points to a vague sense of difference, appropriating and warping scientific language.

It's not pleasant for anyone to realize that they once held bigoted beliefs. But it's worth working through it. The only moral failure as parents is to fall back on defensiveness and ultimately resist updating one's worldview when faced with disturbing truths. When it comes to racism and other forms of prejudice, the impact is what matters, not our intentions nor our own hurt feelings when someone says *Hey, listen, that view you're espousing is bigoted. Here's why.*

Researchers and doctors have long imagined race's impact as a mysterious force that digests real-world circumstances and churns out unequal outcomes across measures of well-being. "There's this idea of a black box," around the concept of race, Tsai tells me on a 2021 phone call. In science, engineering, and computing, a *black box* describes a system with unknown internal functions or mechanisms. In this view, race is also like a black box, an opaque system in which only inputs and outputs are known. People like

Tsai know that there's nothing genetic about racial health disparities. There is "so much preceding evidence that environmental racism, that inequality, that injustice on so many levels, and so many facets, and so many axes" are acting in that system.

Across our institutions, there has been an indolent notion that variation in everything from athleticism to attitude and disposition to disease risk is, at least on a statistical level, a result of biological variation between races. In this delusion, assumed biological differences between races have a function in that black box. There has been intense pushback against these racist ideas for as long as they've existed.

The pushback culminated after World War II when the United Nations Educational, Scientific and Cultural Organization (UNESCO) convened more than a hundred of the world's eminent scientists in Paris in an effort to define race. Their final statement declared race a social construct—traits like temperament, talent, and physiological disposition have nothing to do with race. Their intention was to finally put the question to rest. But the delusions of whiteness proved stubborn. Over a hundred opponents voiced their objections to the UNESCO statement. Among them was British geneticist Kenneth Mather. "I, of course, entirely agree in condemning Nazi race theory, but do not think that the case against it is strengthened by playing down the possibility of statistical differences in, for example, the mental capacities of different human groups," he wrote. But over the last several decades, evidence, including genetic data, has piled up to substantiate UNESCO's assertion.

In a policy statement published in August of 2019, the AAP announced its intention to eliminate race-based medicine, highlighting that race is a social construct and not a biological one, yet "[p]ediatrics as a field has yet to systematically address the influence of racism on child health outcomes and to prepare pediatricians to identify, manage, mitigate, or prevent risks and harms." It manifests in everything from poor pain management for children with appendicitis to undertreatment for asthma.

But the racism that harms kids doesn't only come from health care. It also comes from *social determinants of health*, which are the economic and social conditions that influence well-being. Children in racialized groups not only experience worse health but also tend to have less access to resources like nutritious and desirable food, high-quality education, safe housing and neighborhoods, clean air and water, and freedom from racism and other forms of discrimination.

These forces are in the ether, and they're "multidimensional" as Hardeman and coauthors describe it in a 2022 article published in the journal *Health Services Research*. One of her team's goals is to shed light on how to more accurately and comprehensively unpack how structural racism predicts birth outcomes for residents of Minnesota, where, while infant mortality on the whole is low compared to the US overall, Black infants are twice as likely to die in their first year compared to white infants. "We think of structural racism as a *totality* of racist institutions that support and reinforce each other," Hardeman tells me. Birth inequities have persisted despite increased policy efforts to address social determinants of health. To effectively stamp out the impacts on children and their families, it is first necessary to elucidate the "interconnection between" and the "potential reinforcing effects" of different elements of structural racism to inform policy interventions, the researchers write.

Rather than ranking geographical areas throughout the US as broadly having high, medium, or low structural racism overall, they broke down racism into six distinct yet interconnected validated domains of interest: Black–white residential segregation, educational inequity, employment inequity, income inequity, homeownership inequity, and criminal-justice inequity. They categorized geographic areas in the US with at least 100,000 people based on the different levels of structural racism for each domain. For instance, the researchers observed high education, income, and criminal-justice and low-employment inequities in some areas compared to the national median. Other areas were shown to have high-employment inequities and only moderately high levels of income and criminal-justice inequities. These "intricate interactions among various dimensions of structural racism" had been largely brushed over until Hardeman's team began tackling it.

Hardeman tells me in an email that, growing up in Minneapolis, she "saw from a young age that not everyone in this community is afforded the same opportunities to be healthy." In middle school and high school, she spent many evenings and weekends at dialysis appointments with her grandmother who was going through kidney failure. Her grandmother experienced so much discrimination and indifference from her medical providers that she eventually decided to stop the treatment that was keeping her alive. "At age 16, I lost my grandmother because she was tired of dealing with a health-care system that didn't seem to care about her." Hardeman urges people to think of the data this way: "Basically, a Black birthing person born in Liberia or Somalia is healthier than a Black birthing person born in the US, even if they both currently live in Minneapolis, because spending your entire life experiencing US racism is *bad for your body*." Differences in economic circumstances alone can't explain the gaps in maternal and infant health. "In the US, a birthing person is statistically more likely to have a healthier baby if they are *poor* and *white* than if they are *rich* but *Black*," Hardeman explains in our emails. "Socioeconomic status can't make up" for the effects of "dealing with racism your whole life."

Without accounting for all of the dimensions of structural racism, including but not limited to the six dimensions the 2022 paper parsed, trying to tackle any particular one in a vacuum is like a game of Whac-A-Mole. Solutions to closing a gap in one dimension of structural racism, like educational inequity, can fail to reduce inequity in other dimensions, like criminal-justice inequity. Improving birthing outcomes in a meaningful way requires a more informed and coordinated effort.

The researchers "call for policies" that will "address all dimensions of structural racism and inequities (or as many as possible)" is a concerted way "to level the playing field for generations to come." The authors note that their study used birth data from only one year from a white-majority state where there are more foreign-born Black folks than those born in the US, which may limit how widely its findings can be applied. They recommend that the next steps include studies that look at multistate and longitudinal data. The findings are the first step in elucidating "the totality of ways in which societies foster racial discrimination through mutually reinforcing systems."

While research is ongoing and there's a lot of detail to discern, it's clear that "the cumulative effects of racism wear down on the bodies of racialized people" throughout their lives in a phenomenon known as "the weathering effect," says Hardeman. "The body is literally aging more rapidly due to chronic disadvantage." In 1992, public-health researcher Arline Geronimus proposed the weathering hypothesis that the health of Black women "may begin to deteriorate in early adulthood as a physical consequence of cumulative socioeconomic disadvantage" as an explanation for racial disparities in health. She faced major pushback at the time from those who insisted that the explanation for racial health disparities must be genetic. But since then, evidence has piled up that it's racism, not race, harming health. Racism exerts continuous stress that damages people's bodies on a cellular level from a young age. These studies have looked at various populations, health outcomes, and physiological mechanisms by which weathering leads to adverse health outcomes. One of these is allostatic load, or the cumulative effects of chronic exposure to the roller-coaster of fluctuating hormonal, neural, metabolic, cardiovascular, and immune responses to repeated stressful experiences. Other factors that researchers think play a role in weathering include the effects of racism and poverty on telomere length, inflammation, and epigenetic changes.

It's long been known that the well-being of families directly impacts the well-being of children. It's no different with systemic racism. Everyday discrimination of parents or other caregivers, like negative stereotypes, can impact caregiving abilities and adult mental health, and that hurts kids.

In 2019, the Wisconsin-based nonprofit organization Foundation for Black Women's Wellness (FFBWW) published its "Saving Our Babies" report, in which it engaged the voices of nearly three hundred Black residents of Dane County, which covers Madison and the surrounding Middleton, Fitchburg, Verona, and Sun Prairie. One of the report's conclusions is that it is crucial to address "the whole life well-being of Black families" in addition to specific health-care initiatives to stamp out the disparities in outcomes for babies once and for all. What happens to our kids today—and to their adult family members—affects them cumulatively for life.

Weathering kicks in before birth with the exposure to stress hormones in response to racialized stress during pregnancy and picks up the pace in childhood. Substantial evidence suggests that constant coping with racism and discrimination is a potent activator of the stress response. Years of research have revealed that kids' stress-response systems staying dialed up for long periods takes a toll on developing brains and other organs and systems.

Another undeniable dimension of the racism that affects children starting before infancy is policing. Greater police presence per capita in Black neighborhoods is well-known and can contribute to birth disparities, in large part because it causes weathering. "This is especially true for my home of Minneapolis, where we face an ongoing pattern of racialized violence, surveillance, and murder from Minneapolis Police," says Hardeman.

"The institution of policing in Minneapolis is *bad for community health*. It's bad for birthing people. It's bad for their babies."

Policing was built on racism and white supremacy. In early America, policing was largely about maintaining the hierarchy. Even as policing has evolved, the well-being and property of the privileged class have continued to take precedence over the lives of underprivileged people. In frontier cities like St. Louis, early police terrorized Native Americans in the name of protecting white residents. In 2016, the nonprofit Equal Justice Initiative called police killings of Native Americans "off the charts and off the radar." According to the CDC's fatal-injury data on firearm deaths by police between 2009 and 2019, Native people were 2.2 times more likely to be killed by police than white people.

In the same vein, when slavery was abolished, slave patrols were reimagined into police, and dogs that were traditionally used to hunt down people who had escaped from their enslavers were rebranded as police dogs. Criminalization became a new form of entrapment rooted in capitalism: the carceral tendrils of the state exist to protect assets while swathes of people toil to uphold this system, all while our children grow up too fast. A society that values property over people is by definition unjust. As the fight to dismantle racism in the institution of medicine rages on, the call to abolish policing and prisons has not let up. In the last few decades and especially in the 2020s, though police violence has received increased attention, data reveals that Black people are still killed by police at higher rates than whites in 2023.

Rather than continue to funnel funding to police and prisons, we need to "understand and get rid of the conditions that produce violence in individuals," said the legendary Angela Davis, PhD, an activist, professor, and author who was jailed for over a year in 1970, and who was instrumental in launching the movement to abolish the prison-industrial complex, in a 2021 interview with *Al Jazeera.*

Another undeniable form of oppression that harms children via the policing of racialized people in the US and abroad is institutionalized Islamophobia. "Islamophobia represents a particular type of oppression that is rooted in anti-religious animus and, based on a Muslim's particular background, intersects with anti-Blackness, racism, cultural racism, nationalism, and xenophobia," writes Maha Hilal, PhD, a researcher and organizer dedicated to dismantling the War on Terror and author of *Innocent Until Proven Muslim,* whom I first met when we both attended the same middle school on the west side of Madison. "Islamophobia is maintained and perpetuated by white supremacy, which upholds notions of dichotomous ideological values between the 'West' and Islam." In her work, Hilal raises awareness of how institutionalized Islamophobia is used to dehumanize and violate the fundamental rights of adults and children alike. This dehumanization doesn't only happen in the bowels of Gitmo and via drone strikes, but everywhere. Spaces where children are meant to be protected, like schools and health-care facilities, are no exception. Among the more well-known examples is the 2015 arrest of Ahmed Mohamed, a Black Muslim adolescent in Texas, after he brought a clock that he built himself to school. One of Mohamed's teachers called the police, believing that what he had brought was not a clock but a bomb. He was handcuffed and arrested. The incident was made possible by Countering Violent Extremism, a US government program that's considered a soft counterterrorism tactic. It "has been incredibly successful at normalizing suspicion of Muslims, including youth and children," writes Hilal. Constant heightened surveillance, whether or not it results in being arrested, is traumatic for children.

For yet another way policing harms children, consider the armaments of police departments, like tear gas, an umbrella term for chemicals that specifically activate pain receptors in the eyes, respiratory system, and skin. One of the most widely used chemical crowd-control agents is aerosolized CS gas, which has been described in the literature as a "powdered barb" that attaches to all moist membranes. The 1925 Geneva Protocol categorized tear gas as a chemical warfare agent and banned its use in war shortly after World War I, but it's still legal and harms kids in the United States, even when it's not sprayed directly in their vicinity or right at them—which, to be clear, can and does happen. In South Portland, Oregon, where there have been protests at an ICE facility in a residential neighborhood since 2020, police have regularly used tear gas and other chemical weapons. Families in nearby high-rise apartments have had the substances seep into their homes, where the noxious fallout can linger stubbornly. Over a hundred similar stories played out in cities all across America in the summer and autumn of 2020 alone.

US law-enforcement agencies use what they claim to be scientific rationale to support the continued use of these chemicals. It's no different for the Madison Police Department (MPD), which I consider a hazard to my children and other kids in my city.

Following clashes between Madison Black Lives Matter activists and the MPD in July 2020, a Madison alderperson proposed a resolution to ban the use of tear gas, mace, and impact-projectile devices as crowd-control measures. To some Madisonians, like independent journalist Scott Gordon, the decision should have been a no-brainer. "There are no two ways about it. Get it the fuck done," he wrote in the local publication *Tone Madison* on July 5.

This wasn't only a journalist's opinion. In less direct terms, David Sterken, MD, hospitalist, and faculty member at the UW-Madison School of Medicine, urged the city council in an August 21 email to ban chemical crowd-control agents. He referred to footage of Madison police in full riot gear spraying peaceful protesters on State Street directly in the face with pep-

per spray. Shortly thereafter, the video shows protesters screaming in pain and fear as police shoot tear-gas grenades into the
crowd. I "hope you can all agree that this was not a justifiable
use of chemical agents," he wrote.

"This is an issue of physical harm coming to citizens of your
city at the hands of city employees, so it is your duty to understand it." He referred to several studies that suggest short- and
long-term respiratory harm and an increase in the spread of viral
illnesses, including COVID-19 from the effects of these chemical agents, and pointed out that the American Thoracic Society
called for their moratorium on June 11.

The cops had other ideas. In an email response to Sterken
copied to city council members, Ashley Anderson, MD, medical director for the MPD, took issue with Sterken's rationale.
Among Anderson's objections was Sterken's conclusion about
two studies: a 2013 literature review of three riot-control agents
and a 2014 analysis of long-term effects of tear gases on the respiratory system. Sterken asserted that the studies show that "[t]
ear gas is known to cause a variety of potentially severe short-
term and long-term health effects, including chronic bronchitis,
compromised lung function, and acute lung injury."

In his refutation of Sterken's claim, Anderson quoted from
and dismissed the 2014 study: "This study focuses on subjects
'frequently exposed' to these agents. It is more relevant for [law
enforcement] personnel than for those exposed due to civil un-
rest on an occasional basis."

Anderson's response seemed to remove these conclusions from
crucial context. The full quote from *BMJ Military Health* reads
"In the majority of exposures, significant clinical effects are not
anticipated. The irritant effects can be minimized both by rapid
evacuation from sites of exposure, decontamination and appropriate supportive care."

Greg Gelembiuk, PhD, a scientist researching evolutionary
genomics at UW–Madison who served on the ad hoc City of

Madison police procedure and policy committee in 2019, took issue with Anderson's "quibbling," pointing out that this doctor "is a lone individual, working for the Madison Police Department." Based on their votes, some of these alders were convinced by a doctor employed by the MPD, which is, frankly, pretty unsettling. They took the science that this doctor chose to present as support for their ostensible view that the police need these harmful weapons.

When it comes to the science of tear gas, the fact is that in the real world, people often get stuck and can't flee from the harmful irritants. In his email to the city council, Gelembiuk quoted Dr. Rohini J. Haar, MD, MPH, an emergency physician and health and human-rights researcher at UC Berkeley, who told *Popular Science* that the dangers of tear gas have long been known and "[t]he science is not moving the policy the way it should."

There are no two ways about it. Science has failed to upend the status quo. This isn't a struggle between those who believe science is real and those who don't. It's a function of the ideologies of those with power and their ability to appropriate science to prop up their agendas.

As of this writing, the Madison Common Council did not get it done. At their October 7, 2021, deliberation, with all of this evidence at their disposal, rather than ban tear gas, the city council voted to commission a study from MPD on tear-gas alternatives. That study unsurprisingly found that tear gas "has been critical to successfully resolving those instances in which it has been used[.]"

One commonality between the prevailing views about racism in medicine and in policing is the outsized focus on implicit bias, generally defined as *bias that occurs automatically, unintentionally, or subconsciously*. To combat this form of bias, since 2002, the concept of "cultural competence"—or the knowledge and skills for clinicians to thoughtfully provide treatment to people with diverse cultures and values—has emerged and become increasingly embedded in health-care curricula and training around the world. And, similar to other contexts like law enforcement, implicit-bias training, or programs designed to expose people to their unconscious biases, is becoming a common element of racial equity programs in health care.

But Tiffany Green says implicit-bias training and so-called cultural competence aren't nearly as helpful to birthing people as proponents make them out to be. Instead, Black birthing people need "competent care" period, she explains to me on a phone call in February of 2021. As for implicit-bias training, Green doesn't necessarily think it shouldn't happen, but "we're trying to shepherd state and federal resources for implicit-bias training" when systemic racism is "hiding in plain sight," she says. It doesn't make sense to spend time and resources on implicit bias when there are all of these blatant problems to fix. Green is concerned that poorly executed implicit-bias training can actually lead to resentment in white men—making life harder, not easier, for non-white people. She says that while researchers are working hard to create implicit-bias training, clinics aren't ready to implement them. We still need research to answer several foundational questions about bias and stereotyping, including whether and how they drive disparities in actual outcomes. According to Green, "it's a mess" that these trainings are happening before we get the answers to these questions.

In a May 2021 paper in *Obstetrics & Gynecology*, Green and her coauthors explain that there is currently no evidence that implicit-bias training actually changes how health-care providers treat patients. Ultimately, approaches that center implicit bias ignore "the complex ways that racist practices extend far beyond individual actors and are embedded in organizational processes and our legal and social systems." As an economist who thinks about the scarcity of resources, implicit-bias trainings are "not a good use of resources," she says. "We know that some vague behaviors are associated with implicit bias, but connecting all that to patient outcomes has been really tricky."

Like police officers, there's a lot of talk about doctors and nurses who are bad apples in an otherwise good bunch. Green points me to the Black Maternal Momnibus Act that Congresswoman Lauren Underwood, Congresswoman Alma Adams, and members of the Black Maternal Health Caucus introduced in 2021. The act emphasizes hiring a more diverse perinatal workforce so that Black and other marginalized women are getting culturally competent care. Green recounts "and I'm like, hold up, is the implication here that white people cannot provide competent care?"

The first half of the one bad apple metaphor is often taken out of context in policing and health care to suggest that one or a few corrupt individuals are not representative of the group. The original version of the aphorism—based, by the way, on the science of how apples decay—says the opposite, concluding that rotten apples ruin the entire group: *one bad apple spoils the bunch.* They need to be completely removed; adding fresh new apples doesn't counteract existing rot.

Bad apples are on my mind, so I ask Green if there should be a push to fire racist clinicians who cause tangible harm in the same vein as the push to fire racist cops. "[Y]our point is really good because we're not taking it to the logical conclusion" of removing the bad apples, Green says. "Do I think that we need to increase the number of Black providers? Of course I do." But having Black providers available to all Black patients isn't feasible. Fundamentally, "we need to have a serious conversation about who should be practicing medicine." For instance, if a nurse keeps giving the wrong dosage of medication to a Black patient, "you don't just say, 'Oh well, we need to do a little training,'" Green says.

As if to reinforce what's in clinicians' minds, racism has long been baked into the very algorithms health-care providers use to manage patients. Certain diagnostic and clinical decision-making tools take as their assumption that race is biologically real, adjusting or "correcting" their outputs based on the identified race or ethnicity of a patient. But, just like other studies that analyze spurious observational data from previous studies, the outputs are only as good as their data and assumptions, and the data and assumptions are flawed. For instance, until recently, clinics used a risk calculator that estimates the likelihood that someone will have a successful VBAC, or vaginal birth after a previous Cesarean section, instead of ending up with a repeat C-section. The calculator takes as its fundamental assumption that race and ethnicity are markers of innate differences between people of different races. Along with age, Body Mass Index (BMI), and history of vaginal delivery, this calculator also includes two *yes* or *no* questions: "African-American?" "Hispanic?" If the answer to one or both of those questions is *yes*, the birthing person is automatically given a lower chance of having a successful trial of labor. The result influences whether a doctor recommends trying for a vaginal delivery or opting for a repeat Cesarean. In some cases, the VBAC calculator has been used to prohibit some birthing people from attempting a trial of labor, essentially pushing them into repeat C-sections.

Green chuckles in frustration as we talk about it. "There's no biological reason why either of those things should be linked to the successful trial of labor except for the fact that an observational study found that race and ethnicity were correlated with a successful trial of labor," she says. But other social factors that are correlated with a successful trial of labor don't show up in the calculator, like marital status. When people "think of race as a biological or genetic category, that's how you're going to behave, and that's how these behaviors become institutionalized."

White children don't escape racism's harm, either. I've heard a repeated alarm over the problem of whiteness as an arbitrary "default" or "control group."

In medicine, this can mean accepting what's middling as the standard. On a 2021 phone call, Ruqaiijah Yearby, JD, MPH, the cofounder and executive director of the Institute for Healing Justice and Equity at Saint Louis University, asks me to consider a sports analogy. As a big tennis fan, Yearby says, "Serena is the best." Serena "has been the best, and nobody would look at Anna Kournikova" and say "that's who I want to be." It's "the same thing in the infant mortality realm, you want to try to get to the Serena levels." The issue is that, even though whiteness has retained social and economic advantage in the racialized system overall, white people in the United States don't have the best health outcomes across the board. For instance, "Asian Americans have the best health outcomes when it comes to infant mortality," Yearby points out. Since research to clarify what "actually leads to better health outcomes" in these groups is scant, we aren't able to "figure out" how to achieve the best possible outcomes for everyone. She also stresses that it's not accurate to say that "all Asians" have better outcomes because of the diversity within that group. When looking at groupings outside of race, Yearby points out that overall, infants born to recent immigrants to the United States have a lower risk of mortality across races, though these findings are still preliminary. This is why she is against a "colorblind" approach to medicine because it "ignores the impact of racism on health-care outcomes" and ultimately reinforces injustice. Confronting racism requires unraveling and taking into explicit account the many ways that systemic injustices lead to disparate health outcomes.

As Tsai and her coauthors explained in the October 2020 issue of *The Lancet*, medical research, education, and practices need to intentionally adopt "race-conscious medicine." Racialized clinical decision-making, like medical algorithms, must be carefully replaced by race-conscious alternatives. Instead of biomedical research that links race with disease, race-conscious research will analyze the effects of structural racism. Social race should be tracked in health care and other settings as a way to explicitly contend with racism.

Maybe it's that I'm a medical and health nerd who is also a parent, but I see a direct parallel between the shifts in medicine over time—from racialized to colorblind to race-conscious—and the needed and ongoing shifts in parents' attitudes and in how we raise kids. Outside of medicine, antiracist activists and educators have been pointing out the problem with racial "colorblindness" in society, or the idea that race or ethnicity should be and therefore are irrelevant in interpersonal, social, legal, and other contexts. Antiracist parents have started to learn that it's important to reject colorblind ideology in the behaviors and belief systems we model for our children.

The idea that skin color doesn't matter is a false and misguided ideal. The fact is, skin color is real, even if it's only skin deep. Like so many other Americans who don't have a European skin tone, I can't count how many times I've heard a variation of "I don't care whether you're brown, black, white, yellow, green, or purple," starting in childhood. Listen, folks, there's no other way to say it: always care if someone has turned purple or green. The sentiment can be well-intentioned, but it's counterproductive, and a result of avoidance of the discomfort that comes with interrogating one's own views on race. It's not only okay but necessary to be conscious of our children's skin color because we know that it affects how others perceive them and how they experience the world. As a society, we need to see skin color for countless reasons, including ones as seemingly benign as multinational corporations selling only beige tights or Band-Aids and calling these shades *nude*. If people don't care if someone is purple, green, white, or brown, how are we supposed to get the right match for our makeup, let alone the best dermatological care?

At the same time, being conscious of race doesn't mean that it's okay to comment on race in every setting. For instance, there are more parents with multiracial families than ever, and they have been increasingly speaking out about inappropriate comments and questions they often receive, like "Is this child yours?" or "Are you their nanny?" or "Are they adopted?" There is no appropriate time to ask strangers about their family's multiracial background, but it happens all the time. Never assume anything about someone's racial background. People will share clarifying information if and when they so choose.

When whiteness is the default, the standard to which we hold our society and communities, as Green puts it on a phone call in 2021, "is going to stay basic." In one sense, she feels "frustration that people don't get it, and that we're not moving ahead quickly enough." Like me, Green is "a child of the '80s." Like me, she watched *The Jetsons*. "I don't have a flying car yet," she often vents righteously. "And the reason I don't have a flying car is because we are keeping people from reaching their highest potential," she says. As a society, "we could be doing so much more" for our children. "What could these babies become? What could these birthing parents become if they had the resources?

"When we are racist, when we are ableist, we lose so much, and so from a purely self-interested perspective, I just work because I want a flying car. That's real talk."

History and science shed light on what race—and even ethnicity and ancestry—really is and isn't. People who have lived in the United States are intimately familiar with checking off the demographic boxes for race and ethnicity on paperwork, even when none of them quite capture your identity. I've selected *Asian* for most of my life without considering why. Does something about the continent of Asia define me? More recently, I've encountered the option to check *South Asian*. Would it be more politically accurate if I could write in *India* as the place my ancestors lived? Or am I Tamil, like others who trace their ancestry to the South Indian state of Tamil Nadu, where my parents, grandparents, and their known ancestors before them lived? Or am I a Gounder, a community with a rich culture that originated in Western Tamil Nadu (and, while not considered the highest caste, is a dominant caste that has historically benefited from unearned privileges to the detriment of people of lower castes and *Dalits*, also known as *outcasts*)? Many Americans perceive me to be vaguely brown, often trying to guess my ethnicity (these guesses have run the gamut from Mexican to Dominican to Greek to Black to "dot or feather" to "one of those 9/11 people"). No matter how my kids or I slice our ethnicities, none of it is biologically real.

America as we know it—and its legacies of genocide, slavery, capitalism, the prison-industrial complex, institutionalized Islamophobia, and other forms of oppression—was forged in the fires of racism. The economic and social system of colonial European-Americans required land and labor, which relied on the racialization and dehumanization of African and Native peoples. That forging and honing are evident in the race categories on each US census, which have been in flux from the beginning. Their manifestation decade after decade reflects each era's predominant political view of race. The first census taken in 1790 had only three racial categories: "free whites," "all other free persons," and "slaves." In 2020, the census options were "White," "Black or African-American," "American Indian or Alaska Native," "Asian," "Native Hawaiian and Pacific Islander," or "Some Other Race," with options to provide a detailed identity or pick more than one category.

None of these have ever been biological categories.

In unpacking our beliefs about race as progressive parents, as we did with infant feeding, let's start at the beginning. We know that *Homo sapiens* originated more than 300,000 years ago in Africa and, roughly 60,000 years ago, groups of what we consider modern humans left the continent and populated the Earth. Over thousands of generations, populations who lived farther away from the equator lost melanin in the skin, allowing for sufficient vitamin D production where sunlight was scarce. No fundamental genetic or tissue-deep changes accompanied this surface-level change in the skin color of humans.

Concepts like genetic ancestry and ethnicity have increasingly taken over as stand-ins for race. But even these categories are social constructs, and they're squishier than most people realize.

Racial classification has long used continents as meaningful boundaries, so it's no surprise that race and continental ancestry are often conflated. Many people describe their children as 25% this or 50% that. Despite the booming popularity of direct-to-consumer genetic ancestry tests, which have suggested that your DNA can sort you into roughly continent-based racelike categories, there's nothing about someone's genetic sequence that makes them 98% one ethnicity or 2% another. Geographic regions don't reside in our children's genes.

The results of these consumer ancestry kits are based on self-reported ancestry data from customers known as *reference groups* whose families have a long-known history in some particular place on Earth. The results don't tell someone that their DNA is, say, 30% German. Rather, the individual shares around 30% of their DNA sequence with people whose most recent ancestors were known to have lived within the geographical borders of what we consider Germany.

Everyone gets 50% of their genome from each parent. That also means 50% of each parent's DNA *isn't* passed on to their child. What's included and left out is random.

Before sex cells divide to create sperm and eggs, they undergo a process called recombination, when the chromosomes line up in pairs and swap bits and pieces of genes. After reshuffling, the cells divide, typically cutting the two sets of 23 chromosomes into one set of 23 in each. Each mature egg and sperm has its own slightly unique permuation of DNA. When a sperm and egg merge during fertilization, they form a full human genome.

Everyone is the biological offspring of two parents, each with two biological parents of their own. This means we have four grandparents, eight great-grandparents, sixteen great-great-grandparents, and so on; the number of ancestors in each generation increases exponentially. The reports that come with tests like AncestryDNA and 23andMe provide a somewhat reliable snapshot of where your ancestors lived going back about eight generations, or the generation in which you had roughly a hundred ancestors (that number is 128, but let's call it a hundred for the sake of this explanation). As of this writing, AncestryDNA's data divides the world into over eighty-four global subregions, which it calls *ethnicities*, of Africa, America, Asia, Europe, Oceania, and West Asia, which are then further subdivided based on their available reference data.

Think of each individual's genes as a deck of 50 cards. You got 25 from each parent. If you have a sibling who shares both of your biological parents and isn't your identical twin, they also got a mix of 50 cards, 25 from each parent. Probability dictates that about half of that sibling's 50 cards (25 cards) would be the same cards you received. That's why someone's ancestry results can differ from their own sibling's because their parents' sperm and egg cells all contain different permutations of genetic information from each of their own parents. But that doesn't mean that having a higher percentage ethnicity estimate from, say, France, makes one sibling "more French" than another.

If you go 20 generations back, or around 400 years assuming 20 years per generation, we each have about a million ancestors. Forty generations back, or around a thousand years ago, each one of us has a trillion ancestors. That's far more humans than the approximately 117 billion humans that have ever lived on this planet. It is a statistical certainty that, tens of generations ago, not only do many of your ancestors appear on both your mom's and dad's sides of your family tree, some of those same ancestors also appear on both sides of your favorite celebrity's family tree.

Humanity has always been in geographic flux with groups disseminating, converging, crisscrossing, and backtracking, so pinning down ethnicities on a map is largely a made-up endeavor.

In the deck of cards analogy, copies of the same cards you have—or little pieces of cards that went through the most granulated shredder—are scattered throughout humanity. Nobody has the exact same cards, but there is immense overlap. It gives a whole new meaning to the cultural practice of calling your parents' unrelated friends Auntie and Uncle, because, to some degree, they really are. All strangers are really relatives of varying degrees.

Though ethnicity doesn't reside in our kids' bodies by way of their DNA, the social force of race seeps organ-deep, sometimes in ways that are perhaps as ridiculous as they are appalling. Writing in *Slate* in June of 2021, Tsai exposes yet another tale that reveals the sheer inanity—and inherent violence—in how "racism gets under the skin to jeopardize the health and well-being of Black bodies." Tsai met young Jordan Crowley, then eighteen years old, at the start of the pandemic. He has spoken out about how he was born with only a single shrunken kidney, which has steadily lost function over the years. Tsai writes of knowing firsthand that bad kidney disease is often so deadly "that when an ambulance patch crackles over the radio announcing an incoming sick dialysis patient—'we'll be there in five'—I can feel the whole team tense."

Tsai details that, throughout his childhood, Jordan's biracial mother, Jessica, and his white grandmother, Joyce, were by his side, advocating for the best treatment for him. Jordan's family has been waiting for him to be listed for kidney transplantation. During this stressful process, Jordan and his family were shocked to learn that the medical algorithms his providers were using to assess his kidney health yielded different results for Black and non-Black patients.

A patient's level of kidney disease is assessed partially by an estimate of glomerular filtration rate, or eGFR. Measuring the precise glomerular filtration rate, or GFR, requires particularly costly and time-consuming methods. In 1999, a major study published in the *Annals of Internal Medicine* measured the GFR of more than 1,500 patients to develop a model that could easily predict kidney function using just a rapid blood test and some number crunching—the eGFR. The equation was absorbed into medicine and quickly became a standard of care.

A rate between 90 and 120 is considered normal in someone with two healthy kidneys. In the United States, patients can't be listed for a kidney transplant until their eGFR dips below 20. The eGFR adds a race-specific multiplier to a Black individual's score (and no other race), giving Black patients with kidney disease an inflated score. The equation that calculates eGFR plugs in creatinine levels in the blood, which is an indicator of how well the kidneys are cleaning out the byproducts of normal muscle function. In the 1999 study, the authors observed that overall, the Black patients in their dataset had higher levels of creatinine in their blood. Based on poorly interpreted observational data, the authors surmised this was likely because "on average, Black persons have higher muscle mass than white persons." Instead of interrogating that false, racist assumption about muscle mass and race, they added a race-based coefficient that inflates the eGFR of patients "if Black."

Jordan's estimated GFR "depends on how you interpret" the fact that he is biracial. "Jordan's doctors decided he is Black, meaning he doesn't qualify," Tsai writes. "So now, he has to wait."

More daunting is that researchers are finding that in some situations, simply removing race measures from clinical prediction, however well-meaning, could actually be worse for health equity. Just like you shouldn't simply pull out a knife that's impaled someone, undoing the racism built into clinical tools isn't as easy as hitting Ctrl+Z. The VBAC calculator and eGFR equation have been replaced in some practices by new versions that remove race and ethnicity as risk factors. But this is hardly a fix for inequity for birthing people. The VBAC calculator cannot account for racism's role in a birthing person's lived experience. "While there has been a movement over the past few years to reconsider and remove race as an indicator for VBAC success, we still have a long way to go," Hardeman warns.

Consider sickle cell disease (SCD), a common inherited blood disorder, and sickle cell trait, or the allele that causes SCD when inherited from both parents. It's widely believed that SCD—a condition present at birth, and the poster child for the idea of genetic racial difference—is most common in Black people. This pervasive belief can mislead us in a sneaky way.

SCD is a Mendelian or single-gene disease, meaning it's caused by a mutation in just one gene that's involved in making hemoglobin, or the oxygen-transporting proteins in red blood cells. Babies who inherit two normal alleles—or an HbA/HbA genotype—won't have sickle cell disease. Neither will one with one HbA and one HbS. Their blood circulation isn't usually severely affected because the normal HbA compensates enough for blood to flow fairly efficiently. These individuals are considered *carriers* of sickle cell trait because they have a 50% chance of passing on that HbS allele to each offspring. Around 1.5% of all newborns are *carriers* of this trait. Those with SCD have two copies of HbS. They can't make the normal protein; their phenotype is red blood cells that are crescent-shaped instead of round and smooth, so they're destroyed faster than healthy blood cells, leading to pain, tissue damage, potential respiratory issues, and shortened life expectancy. The better the condition is managed from birth, the better the quality and span of life.

Black babies born in the US are twenty-three times more likely to be carriers of sickle cell trait compared to white babies. That statistic makes it seem like, yeah, there is a fundamental genetic difference between races at work. But there isn't. Kids of all skin tones, including white kids, can have mutant hemoglobin alleles. And plenty of Black people have two normal ones. What *is* at work here are recent evolutionary phenomena that acted on segments of humans in tandem with even more recent artificial phenomena: transatlantic slavery.

The vast majority of the millions of humans who were kidnapped and shipped across the Atlantic between 1525 and 1866 were taken specifically from West Central Africa. Proximity to the equator influenced the flora and fauna of geographical regions, including insects and the diseases they carry. Even though they usually don't experience the symptoms and harms of full-blown sickle cell disease, carriers' hemoglobin is just different enough to prevent the parasite that causes malaria from infecting and taking over the bloodstream. From an evolutionary standpoint, the benefit of resistance to this age-old disease in places where it's been endemic for ages began to outweigh the detriments of SCD, at least in terms of reaching reproductive age and having offspring. In this way, over time, sickle cell trait became more common where malaria is endemic because resistance to the disease provided an evolutionary advantage where the disease had long circulated, including parts of Europe. The fact is, SCD happens in people of all skin colors, and at the highest rates in those whose ancestors came from South and Central America, sub-Saharan Africa, parts of the Middle East, Italy, Greece, India, and Southeast Asia. Black Americans who are descended from enslaved people largely came from parts of the African continent where malaria has been endemic, but people descended from ancestors in the southern and northern parts of Africa don't have particularly high rates of the disease at all.

"In the United States, these nuances were lost purely for demographic reasons. Many white Americans tend to be of European extraction, where sickle cell anemia is rare, and Black Americans tend to have West African roots, where it's more common, so it came to be seen as a 'Black disease,'" wrote Saini in *Superior.* "Once viewed this way, it reinforced existing assumptions about essential differences between Blacks and whites. Two independent facts began to align in people's minds. First, that there may be different genes determining health according to race. Second, if Black people suffer illness and death at higher rates than white people, could this then be genetic?"

Among other things that tie parents together is that we aren't only worried about our kids' well-being in childhood. We're trying to set them up to live their best lives for as long as possible. External forces constantly impact phenotype in ways that scientists are still teasing out, even with single-gene diseases like SCD. In the US, sickle cell patients who receive competent care starting in infancy fare better in the long term. Alas, once the white scientific establishment wrongly deemed it a Black disease, they widely dismissed and stereotyped these patients as *sicklers*, regularly accusing them of faking pain to score drugs. The mistreatment from clinicians leads some to avoid care for SCD altogether, increasing the risk of life-threatening complications. As two MDs noted in a 2020 perspective article in the *New England Journal of Medicine* about racism and sickle cell disease, there has been a chilling effect on resource allocation: cystic fibrosis, for instance, is similar to SCD in terms of being a life-threatening, inherited, single-gene disease, but it receives more attention because it hasn't been labeled a *Black disease*. The white privilege inherent in biomedical science and medicine is reflected in the disparate attention to these two diseases. Although cystic fibrosis affects one-third fewer Americans than SCD, it receives an estimated seven to eleven times the amount of research funding per patient. As a result, the Food and Drug Administration has approved four medications for sickle cell and fifteen for cystic fibrosis.

It's hard to pin down what we can do, if anything, to protect kids against racism. Racism is so multidimensional that it requires far more insight than any one expert in the vast arena of parenting-related disciplines could ever contain in their mind.

All I can do is share what I've gleaned over the years as a parent and journalist covering parenthood, health, and the fight for justice.

We need to take any opportunity to undermine race in our parenting, professional, community, or activist roles. The idea that racial groups have distinct tissues, bones, behaviors, and proclivities is an infection in our collective psyche. "The thing to remember is that kids are already making sense of race and biology, but with no guidance," as Brian Donovan, the senior science education researcher at the Humane Genetics Research Lab, told the *New York Times* in 2019.

While supporting the proliferation of more nuanced genetics education, an education that moves beyond Mendel, we can also undermine the idea that race is genetic in everyday interactions with other parents and kids. Jennifer Noble, PhD, a psychologist with over twenty years of advocacy work in the mixed-race community and over fifteen years of clinical experience, emphasizes that thinking of ethnicity as a matter of "fractions" is misguided. Pushing back against the concept of racial essentialism, she argues, is important as a parent. In a series of messages in 2022, I share with Noble that it's amazing to me that, "just a few years ago" my spouse and I would have described our kids as "a quarter Jewish, half Indian" and a quarter Croatian and other ancestries. Funnily enough, the Historical and Biographical Album of the Chippewa Valley, Wisconsin (1891–1892) describes one of my kids' ancestors, known as Mary Ross Quaderer, as follows: "Among the earliest settlers of Barron County is [John Quaderer, farmer and lumberman], whose name will be handed down to posterity as one who has always been a friend of the poor and needy, and who has done much toward the upbuilding of his county and town." On "January 14, 1872, he married Miss Mary Ross, a half-breed Chippewa Indian," it continues, "and to them were born four children."

Now the idea that my kids are half this or a quarter that

seems as morally and scientifically preposterous and harmful as the idea of any human being a *half-breed*, and I shudder to think how benign I believed the notion that they're *half* or *a quarter* anything to be. In nature, there have never been pure ethnicities to mix. We need to tell our children the truth: ancestry is so much more than DNA. Holidays and traditions like Chinese New Year, Deepavali (Diwali), Dia de los Muertos, Eid, Oktoberfest, and Hanukkah aren't in our DNA, they're in our minds and memories. Neither are foods like tamales, jollof rice, fry bread, sushi, pho, challah, and idli. Neither are languages, nor are lands. When we pass down these customs and places to our children, they're not transmitted via blood but via the hearts, minds, stories, and love of generations. This is what makes them beautiful and worth embracing.

If a form requests that parents check only one box for their child's ethnicity or race, or to choose one option for the so-called primary race, if you have the bandwidth to do so, "write the email" challenging the premise of the question. "Silence won't make a difference," Noble tells a parent in a 2023 social-media exchange. Percentages can never describe who our children are. Genes are not our children's destinies.

To "people that are raising young humans in a world that might not change as fast as we want it to," it's worth teaching your kids that "they can always understand someone else's experience and treat them better," says Elmikashfi. We can all accept that it's okay for people to point out when someone's view is wrong.

Parents also need to cultivate their circles thoughtfully. Hong says that, for too many progressive parents, especially white parents, "their circles of influence" have "provided the privileges" and "the safety of not feeling uncomfortable." Talking about race "should be more demanding." We need to widen our circle and surround ourselves with people who challenge us and be willing to go through those conversations despite discomfort. It's not the end of the world if someone points out that a view or action is racist.

Normalizing "being wrong" for your kids doesn't only apply to gender, sexism, misogyny, and homophobia but to race and racism, too. Owning up to a mistake is not an admission of guilt or a character flaw but just another antiracist practice. Acknowledge to children that, while it's natural to feel discomfort when you realize that you were wrong, working through that discomfort is worthwhile and the opposite of shameful.

We need to work to teach our children to share power by setting an example. Everyone "on this planet, in this country, relative to someone else, we are always going to have power," says Elmikashfi. "Some people have power and some people don't in certain ways."

What keeps racism's wheels turning is people with the power to upend the status quo who fail to act, or who hoard money, power, and influence. In any given situation, for those with the bandwidth, we can actively exercise our power to oppose racism. Sometimes, this means ceding or spreading power. As Green puts it, "think about whether you need to lead the efforts or you need to support the efforts." If you benefit from white or other racial privileges, think about how you can support or fund the work that people without those privileges are doing to dismantle it, and then follow through with doing so. Antiracism amounts to a series of choices that we have to keep on making every day.

That starts with being willing not only to talk about race with our kids, but to teach children that it's okay to experience hard feelings and sit in the discomfort of talking about race. As Ibram X. Kendi puts in his 2022 book *How to Raise an Antiracist*, the tension between "outward optimistic denial and inward fear" about race and racism within ourselves as caregivers applies to how we approach teaching our children. "Caregivers want to believe, optimistically, that their children don't need to learn about it. But that belief is often driven by a fear—the fear of having to confront the troubling truth."

The problem is that "we convince ourselves that it is better for our children if we don't teach them about racism." But the truth is we often put off these conversations and "claim it is about protecting our children when it is really about protecting ourselves." Some parents have performed mental acrobatics, anything to be able to deny that racism will touch their child, anything to keep insisting that their child will be unaffected by the racism around them.

It can be helpful to think of antiracism as an ongoing series of parenting choices and discussions with our children. No matter who we are, as Kendi puts it, "racist and antiracist don't describe who a person is in an absolute sense; they describe us from moment to moment, based on what we're doing and why we're doing it." Racist and antiracist are "not identities, not reflections of what's in anyone's bones or heart." He points out that "countless individuals advocate for both racist and antiracist policies at different times."

To truly "be antiracist, we must admit the times we are being racist" he writes. "They must acknowledge the gravity of the emergency—our society is dangerously racist—and the gravity of their power—I can still raise a child to be antiracist."

Since racism is an emergency that's all around us, it can make sense to treat it that way as a parent. We are continuing to figure out how our family can do our part in fighting against it when we can, while also doing our best to protect ourselves when we have to.

The purpose of *representation* in any decision-making body is to maximize the marginalized viewpoints in the work of ultimately achieving true equity and justice for all children and the adults in their lives. *Diversity* is often framed as a seat at the table next to the powers that be, but it should never be just one or two seats. When it comes to racism, *justice* can look like unseating those with relative racial privilege. In other words, when a decision is relevant to a minoritized group, then the table needs to largely or solely seat people from that group. For instance, when policies to counter anti-Asian and –Pacific Islander hate are on the table, not one or two Asians but multiple AAPI folks are calling the shots. If the decisions and policies are about Black people, Black individuals are at the helm. If the lands and health of specific Indigenous and Native peoples are on the agenda, then these peoples should be at the helm. If broad racial equity is on the line, that table needs to seat a representative set of people. *Inclusion* is ensuring that all of these voices are heard and empowered. When urgency is warranted in the fight for justice for children, accept that those fighters may need to seize and chop up the table for kindling to warm those in immediate need. Sometimes, we have to make the call to either help them or get out of their way.

At the same time, remember that non-white people can and do buy into white supremacy and that people of any race can and do choose to uphold inequity, especially when it increases their perceived proximity to power. Beware that any entity can appropriate, leverage, and capitalize on the language and rhetoric of social-justice movements without demonstrating a commitment to those values, including antiracism. Be vigilant.

There are tangible, albeit limited, ways to empower our families against racism in health care.

In a 2023 email exchange with Dr. Maria Trent, MD, MPH, one of the lead authors of the 2019 AAP policy statement, I ask how to find pediatricians and other providers who have done the work to "address and ameliorate the effects of racism" on children.

"There is no listing of individuals who have decided to incorporate the AAP recommendations," Trent shares, adding that she believes that the volume of downloads of the policy statement is promising, though they do not have data on how many have

read and understood this policy statement, let alone done anything to implement it. Providers should be "patient-centered"
and "family-engaged," Trent shares. Red flags include a doctor or nurse who is "dismissive" or shows "discomfort and lack
of openness when patients or parents share concerns about discrimination" or "differential treatment."

The AAP also urges pediatricians to integrate evidence-based
screening tools that incorporate valid measures of racism into
clinical practice. But there's also no straightforward, standard,
transparent way to determine if a practice has done so.

Hardeman says that "Black people know when they are experiencing racism. They know when they are disrespected, ig-
nored, and mistreated. They know when it happens during their
daily lives, and they know when it happens within health-care
systems."

It's not always immediately clear, though. Trent explains that,
although "[p]atients and their parents are excellent in recognizing their discomfort" in the face of "disrespect" in the clinical setting, it can still be "hard to pinpoint" racism until after a
parent has "processed the visit, unless there is a clear personally
mediated adverse experience in the office." She suggests making
note of whether the clinician uses "listening behaviors associated with effective patient-centered communication." Some of
these behaviors include making space for the patient and parent to talk, asking open-ended questions, and confirming that
they understand.

Lisa Peyton-Caire, a longtime advocate for Black maternal and
child health justice in Wisconsin and the founder of FFBWW,
encourages folks to go to appointments prepared, stressing that
it can be a matter of life or death. This is why she advocates for
patients, especially Black women, to avoid going to appointments alone if they can help it. Take a family member or friend
as an advocate, even a layperson, to act as a "witness" and to

make note of questions and answers, she tells me on a call in July of 2022.

"Most people don't think that they should have to take someone to the doctor and you would like to believe that you wouldn't have to," says Peyton-Caire. In addition to racism, "class and income and everything is operating at the same time," she explains. "Social class and ranking and people's perceptions" affect "how you're addressed as a health-care consumer, how people think you can interpret what they're saying, their tone, and how they're saying it to you." Her organization regularly hears from Black women who say that a clinician was "talking to me so slowly like I was a five-year-old, and it was offensive" because they had just addressed "the person next door" like they're "an intelligent adult." This ties into stereotypes about Black women's "intelligence and our ability to understand complex information," says Peyton-Caire. Someone "could be living in a mansion with a six-figure income and none of it matters." She points to the case of Shalon Irving, PhD, MPH, MS, CHES, an epidemiologist with the CDC who dedicated her life to understanding how structural racism, intersectionality, trauma, and violence over lifetimes contribute to health disparities. Irving suffered a sudden cardiac arrest at home in 2017 just three weeks after giving birth to her daughter, hours after yet another visit to her medical providers, where she knew she was in medical distress, and where she pleaded for help. She complained that her providers dismissed her pleas, as they had before.

"It didn't matter that Shalon had a dual PhD," write the authors of a 2022 article in *Health Affairs* honoring her legacy. Among those authors are Dr. Irving's young daughter, Soleil, and mother, Wanda, who is raising her grandchild. "It didn't matter that she had an MPH from the top-ranked school of public health in the world. It made no difference that she was a lieutenant commander in the US Public Health Service, was an officer in the world-renowned Epidemic Intelligence Service, was a highly respected epidemiologist at the CDC," they write. "She was still a Black woman." The authors explain that, journalists' inquiries into the story later identified what they call "a string of missed opportunities" to take Shalon's case seriously. "We believe it was due to the covert bias of her providers," they write. "This bias, fueled by structural racism, is the root cause of disparities in health care."

Patients "should be able to have a clear conversation with their provider/clinician" about whether race is being considered in "any clinical decision-making (whether an algorithm or calculator is used or not)," Hardeman says.

"You must go prepared to ask for clarification of any terms or information you do not understand, and it is absolutely imperative that you get those answers," Peyton-Caire urges. It is the provider's duty to "go that extra mile," with each and every question or concern. When clinicians "don't go the extra mile" it is a "substandard quality of care." If a provider is unable to explain things in plain language, they have shown their inability to communicate effectively. The burden should be on them to convey a medical assessment in clear terms.

It's also worth keeping an eye on our doctors' notes. A 2022 study published in *Health Affairs* that looked at doctors' notes between January 2019 and October 2020 for over 18,000 patients at an academic medical center in Chicago found that Black patients, including children, had over twice the odds of having at least one negative descriptor in their patient history and notes. On the whole, it's unnerving that parents need to stay on our toes and enlist friends to protect kids against racism in health care. But for now, it's the best we have.

Meanwhile, we can't settle. Structural racism "is a *fixable* problem, and *everyone* has a role to play in the solutions," says Hardeman. "[S]ometimes the problems we face seem overwhelming. Sometimes you just want to grow numb in the face of racism, tragedy, and heartbreak. But we keep fighting because the work of antiracism is *fueled by love*. And when we are fueled by love, we find where we can make a positive impact and *do the work*."

Remember that to practice antiracism, kindness isn't the same as being nice. When faced with the choice between being nice and confronting racism, confront racism.

5

case studies in parenting with feminism: bodily autonomy, ableism, and fatphobia

I channeled a most ancient attitude the night before my first baby's due date, thinking what pregnant people have thought for countless generations: "Hurry up because I'm done being your vessel, and it is closing time, my baby." As if by my command, my water broke at two in the morning in our second-floor condo overlooking a snow-covered cornfield. Nestled on the other side of that field was the elementary school our children would attend a few years later. Heeding the triage nurse's instructions over the phone, we tried to rest for a few hours before heading to the hospital, though the attempt to fall back asleep proved futile for me. By late morning, with no sign of labor starting on its own, I was offered Pitocin, a drug that induces contractions. If the window between the water breaking and the birth was too long, the nurse explained, the risk of infection would rise because the rupture of the gestational sac allows entry for infection. I understood what all of this meant and agreed to the planned course of action. This would be my final opportunity to make a truly informed choice about this birth. Years later, I would realize that, as for the right to choose, it's not just whether and when someone carries out a pregnancy. It's about so much more, including how someone gives birth.

When the Pitocin kicked in and labor started, it took a few hours for my cervix to dilate ten centimeters. Eventually, I had around an hour of pain relief and rest after receiving epidural anesthesia. Finally, it was time to push. The nurses were kind and encouraging, but after over two painful hours of pushing to no avail—all while they encouraged me to keep going, that I was doing great, that this process was worthwhile—I had a nagging feeling that the staff were gaslighting me, even if they didn't realize it. The top of my baby's head had barely budged.

Meanwhile, there were signs of fetal distress, including an abnormal heart rate. That evening, it became clear that she needed to be delivered right away. The doctor strongly advised a forceps delivery. I could hardly consider the implications. I was distraught and unable to think of much more than putting an end to it, so I nodded and breathlessly said yes to the procedure. Only in retrospect did I recall that all day no one had brought up the possibility of using forceps until just then. Before that day, health-care providers seemed to largely gloss over the potential for forceps or vacuum-assisted delivery, known together as assisted vaginal delivery.

Forceps, which the American College of Obstetricians and Gynecologists (ACOG) describes as looking "like two large spoons," are used when there are concerns about the baby's heart-rate patterns during labor, the head stops moving down the birth canal after pushing for "a long time," or if a medical condition prevents safe or effective prolonged pushing. One of the stated main benefits of assisted vaginal delivery with forceps or vacuum is to avoid Cesarean delivery, as a C-section "is major surgery and has risks, such as heavy bleeding and infection." That's true. What's too often overlooked is that vaginal deliveries also come with risks.

My vague understanding on that frigid January day was that forceps are used extremely rarely. I gleaned this understanding from a couple of brief conversations with my doctor and other providers during my pregnancy. I learned from friends, family, childbirth classes, and the internet that our bodies are "designed" to give birth, and that birth is a natural process that should be trusted. Nearing my due date, I was twenty-eight years old, and all in all, my pregnancy was considered low risk. Everything I learned gave me the false impression that vaginal birth should work out just fine.

Jesse still recalls his horror at the sight of the glinting forceps, which I glimpsed only fleetingly. My epidural had worn off, and I went temporarily insane with pain when the surgeon positioned the tool around my baby's head. Even with the help of the surgeon wielding the forceps, my nurse urged me to push. I remember saying I couldn't. The nurse replied, "Look at me. This is my worried face. You have to give a big push!" So I summoned a burst of energy and pushed while the doctor skillfully maneuvered her instrument, guiding this creature to the light. My mind was no longer in my head the moment she was born. "Look at your baby," the nurse urged gently. I heard her, but the words didn't register. She repeated, "Look at your baby!" I mustered the will to turn my head. My first glimpse of her is forever etched in my mind: primordial and painfully beautiful, the 6-lb, 9-oz being emerged with the umbilical cord looped twice around her neck and with what's called a *true* (tightly pulled) knot. I observed my own mind as it recalibrated.

Despite the mental and physical trauma, I would do it all again and am thankful to those doctors and nurses because that baby is a nerdy, creative, cherished, chatty seventh-grader as of this writing. Fortunately, I healed up relatively well. I had another vaginal delivery in 2013, which was drastically different:

I pushed for about forty-five minutes, and it was gratifying to feel steady progress with every push.

Knowing what I know now, I can't say whether I would have opted for a C-section for my daughter's delivery, but I do think that people should discuss in advance which procedure to use in the event of an emergency. That choice should be informed by a more extensive lay understanding of potential risks of all options in the weeks before birth. I don't blame my care providers for using forceps, but I'm disturbed that I agreed to a serious medical procedure without fully understanding the implications. An informed choice would have involved explaining far earlier on in the process what a forceps birth is really like and a frank explanation of the risks of this procedure. My experience, and hearing about the experiences of dozens of others who had their own traumatic childbirths, opened my eyes to the lack of fully informed consent in obstetrics.

I've learned that a big part of the problem is, yet again, biological essentialism about people who can get pregnant. Our ability to not only endure pain, short-term and lifelong physical reconfiguration, and sacrifice but to do so without question is a fallacious measure of so-called womanhood and femininity. This is the same essentialism, often paired with religious justifications, that led to the Supreme Court's decision to overturn *Roe v. Wade*, and exacerbates the horrific consequences of increasing restrictions on abortions and reproductive health care in recent decades.

When we are truly empowered, we avail ourselves of our right to bodily autonomy. We can actively choose whether or not to use various medical and technological advances. To empower us, the establishment should provide all of the relevant information about any parenting-related decision in a comprehensive, accurate, and accessible way. It should treat us like autonomous beings with the capacity to understand our options when it comes to something as physically and mentally life-altering as creating and bringing an entire human into the world.

Humans have a uniquely rough time giving birth. And no matter how someone gives birth, pregnancy, labor, and delivery permanently alter the body. The prevailing discourse around C-sections is that most of them are unnecessary. Since 1985, the global health-care community has considered 10–15% of births to be the ideal rate of Cesareans on a population level to minimize maternal and infant mortality. In much of the world, including the US, the rate has surpassed 30%, and that's concerning to some stakeholders. The message is clear: You don't want a C-section if you can help it. Women were *designed* to give birth. You just have to *believe in your body*. Like many millions of birthing parents, the messaging had me striving to avoid one, the idea being that, similar to formula-feeding, needing a C-section means you failed.

Reasons for a Cesarean section have typically fallen into two buckets. Some are scheduled ahead of time because of known problems with the placenta or umbilical cord, a breech baby, or other conditions that would make a vaginal delivery particularly dangerous. In other cases, doctors perform C-sections when something goes wrong during an attempted vaginal delivery, like when labor doesn't progress or there are signs of distress. At least, that's how it's supposed to go, but research suggests that doctors sometimes do C-sections for convenience, higher insurance payouts, or to avoid malpractice charges for not doing a C-section if something goes wrong during an attempted vaginal birth. Whether or not a C-section happens is in large part at the discretion of the doctor in charge, and there's no precise formula for when, exactly, a doctor should do one. We also know that, in the US, racism that's built into obstetrics means that Black women are more likely to end up with a medically unnecessary C-section than white women.

In addition to those two buckets, there's a smaller but potentially growing third category: maternal request or "elective" Cesareans, when someone chooses to forgo vaginal birth even when attempting one wouldn't be contraindicated. On a population level, the outcomes for *unplanned* C-sections are worse than with vaginal births. Bad outcomes are associated with C-sections, but that's in large part because something urgent precedes most C-sections.

There are limited data on C-sections by request without a medical indication, which are thought to happen in around 1–2% of US births. One issue with the data is that complications in those with planned, nonemergency C-sections are often reported together with emergency cesareans.

C-sections don't deserve their reputation as something to avoid at all costs. More and more parents, researchers, and doctors in the US and around the world have been championing the right of all pregnant people to weigh the pros and cons, which vary from person to person, of both modes of birth and arrive at an informed choice. The medical community is still wrapping its heads around *my body, my choice* in this context, or as a 2019 statement from the American College of Obstetricians and Gynecologists put it, Cesarean delivery on maternal request, which accounts for around 2.5% of US births, "is not a well-recognized clinical entity." It also stated that "available information that compared the risks and benefits of Cesarean delivery on maternal request and planned vaginal delivery does not provide the basis for a recommendation for either mode of delivery." In other words, there isn't evidence to suggest that planned Cesareans are particularly bad.

ACOG suggests that providers have a conversation with patients interested in choosing a Cesarean without a medical reason, but actually getting one can be an uphill battle. "[T]here seems to be a lot of respect for a woman's right to choose whether or not to proceed with a pregnancy, but not a lot of respect for the decisions that go along with the choice to proceed," Janice

Williams, a mother of two in Toronto who had an unwanted vaginal birth in 2010, told me in a 2021 message. Though her obstetrician agreed to a planned Cesarean in her third trimester, Williams ended up giving birth vaginally with no epidural because there was no anesthesiologist available. The experience led her to cofound the Cesarean by Choice Awareness Network (CCAN), a social-media group where people commiserate and share resources around choice in the mode of delivery. One of the network's goals has been to facilitate connections with doctors who respect their patients' right to choose, says Williams. "We've made great strides when it comes to respecting choice and having better communities of support."

Heidi Brown, MD, assistant professor of Female Pelvic Medicine and Reconstructive Surgery at the University of Wisconsin-Madison, whose research focuses on improving access to effective treatments for pelvic-floor disorders, told me in a 2021 email that "[w]hile pregnancy is associated with an increased risk of pelvic-floor disorders irrespective of mode of delivery, labor and vaginal delivery, especially with forceps, do damage the pelvic floor in ways that planned Cesarean delivery without labor do not." Brown shared that she decided to have a C-section with her first delivery. One reason was that she was thirty-six years old, and it was her first baby—research suggests that older first-time mothers may have a harder time giving birth vaginally. Pelvic-floor disorders also run in Brown's family, which put her at higher risk of developing one with a vaginal delivery. She also planned to have one more baby at the most. Each Cesarean increases the risk of problems with the placenta and uterine rupture, so it's especially important for people who think they may give birth more than twice to consider these risks.

None of this is to say that anyone who thinks labor and vaginal delivery sound unappealing should automatically opt out. But it's not too much to ask doctors to talk respectfully and clearly about options and individual risk factors. "I think it is a disservice not to have a conversation with a patient," Moeun Son, MD, MSCI, who practices in Connecticut and cares for those with higher-risk pregnancies, told me over the phone in 2021. After that conversation, many people will decide to try a vaginal delivery after all, but for some, avoiding the experience of vaginal birth and the potential complications is "the most important thing to them," or "they have had a really bad delivery before, and they really want to avoid that in a subsequent delivery," a preference that she considers "reasonable." Son also explained that doctors aren't obligated to do a Cesarean that isn't medically indicated, in which case "the right thing to do is just refer you to a physician who is willing."

It's important to note that, in recent years, the so-called optimal C-section rate of 10–15% has come into question. In a 2015 study published in the *Journal of the American Medical Association*, researchers looked at births in World Health Organization member countries in 2012 and found that "Cesarean delivery rates of up to approximately 19 per 100 live births were associated with lower maternal or neonatal mortality and concluded that the "[p]reviously recommended national target rates for Cesarean deliveries may be too low."

When I turned to the Searses' advice in that thick *Baby Book*, with its promotion of a healthy attachment between mother and baby, I didn't realize how very Eurocentric, misogynistic, and hetero- and cisnormative it was. With its origins in the series of papers by psychologist and psychiatrist John Bowlby published between the late 1960s and early 1980s, attachment theory hinges on the idea that healthy relationships must develop within a mother–child dyad, or, as the Sears family authors have called it, a "biological pair," primarily in the first year of a child's life. Attachment theory stems from a Western middle-class perspective in which the nuclear family is seen as the essential center of a child's existence and ignores the many communal and extended family-oriented ways of childrearing in the world. The notion pervades the modern parenting psyche and informs culture, social work, research, policy, and the law. The notion that good caregivers must form this type of attachment may fuel unjustified intervention or separation by child protective services when used to judge a parent's caregiving abilities, among other harms.

For generations, people have internalized the idea of *mother's intuition*. It has been used to obscure the truth about parenthood. There is no sex or gender to the warm, heartbreaking, existential connection, affection, and love that a caregiver develops for a child. Gestating and birthing a human physically changes people, but so does being a partner to someone who gives birth. Breastfeeding, which some gender-nonconforming people call chestfeeding, can release warm, fuzzy chemicals in the body. But so do other forms of nurturing and closeness with an infant, like bottle-feeding, holding, cuddling, or sniffing the tops of their heads as they rest on your shoulder. Studies suggest that adults of all genders who take on daily caregiving and engage closely with babies go through cell-deep changes. Testosterone and cortisol levels decrease, and oxytocin, estrogen, and prolactin levels surge in parents, whether or not they've given birth, promoting bonding, love, and devotion. Neuronal pathways undergo transformations when an adult is tasked with the care of an infant. We also know that adults can form intense emotional bonds with older children who aren't infants. Foster parents, adoptive parents, and others who are not so-called biological parents (in terms of haploid genomic contribution) still form their own hormonal and brain-based biological connections that forever change them. We all have some form of intuition about our children that we can feel in our guts.

The bottom line is that the idea of *mother's* intuition or instinct reduces people who can get pregnant to ostensibly innate biological functions, perpetuates a sexist division of labor, and convinces boys, men, and others without uteri that they aren't hardwired for nurturing. There is no truth to the notion that only biological mothers can achieve an arbitrary apex of parenthood. Devoting ourselves to our children can be a great thing, but no particular gender is more wired to do so. Testaments to adoptive love abound in pop culture, like the Kents' love for Clark, Uncle Phil's love for Will, or Matthew Cuthbert's love for Anne Shirley. This kind of love doesn't only happen in movies, TV, and books. It's real and it's as ordinary as it is precious. We all have the right to devote as much time to our children as they need and as our hearts desire. That capitalism, oppression, family separation, and incarceration have stolen time between parents and children is an atrocious blot on the well-being of children.

Along with breaking away from biological essentialism, parenting with feminism is about intersectionality as a practice of radical inclusion. Whiteness, cisnormativity, and heteronormativity aren't the only dehumanizing defaults or control groups that have upheld a deleterious standard. Across society, ableism, or discrimination and prejudice against people with disabilities, also systematically favors people without disabilities to the detriment of everyone else. In the prevailing ableist view, those who exist, think, act, perform tasks, and navigate the world in prescribed ways are *normal*, while those who deviate from the norm are inherently deficient. In effect, the mistaken assumption that supposedly most people fit this default upholds inequity that harms children.

People with disabilities have been called the "largest minority." Globally, over a billion people are estimated to be living with disabilities. Data from the 2019 American Community Survey suggest that over three million children in the United States had a disability that year, with American Indian and Alaska Native children having the highest reported rate of all groups. The separation of children with disabilities into different classrooms or schools is a stark example of how oppression thrives when swathes of humanity are relegated to the fringes, out of sight, out of mind. It is taken as justification to ignore children's needs.

Disability inclusion is key in all diversity, equity, and inclusion efforts. It's about more than merely encouraging participation. Transportation, public facilities, education, employment, and high-quality health care are the bare minimum—the floor, not the ceiling. The end goal of inclusion is for disabled people to be as unfettered as anyone else. It means that everyone gets to be their most expansive and authentic selves.

There's no one definition for *disability* which includes a variety of acute and/or chronic conditions that present challenges with participation in society and the larger world. These include challenges with hearing, vision, cognition, mobility, self-care, and independent living. Note that, increasingly, both person-first language, like *person with autism* or *people with disabilities* and identity-first language, like *autistic person* and *disabled person* are considered appropriate based on someone's preferences and other factors. In the 1970s, people-first language emerged as a way to reject demeaning language and emphasize that disability is only one element of an individual's identity. Eventually, people-first language became a "baseline" that was "codified into the way that we write grants and for federal funding," says Imani Barbarin, a disability-rights advocate who writes from the perspective of a Black woman with cerebral palsy, on a December 2021 panel about ableism. "So you'll find a lot of people who are older disabled people, or a lot of people who are outside of the disability community utilizing person-first language." But "people who were born around the '90s and later generally use identity-first language" as a way to say "I don't need to remind you that I'm a person first, you should already know," she explains.

Awareness of disabilities and ableism has risen since 1990 with the passage of the Americans with Disabilities Act (ADA), a federal civil-rights law that officially prohibits discrimination against people with disabilities in everyday activities. Also in

1990, the Individuals with Disabilities Education Act replaced the 1975 Education for All Handicapped Children Act, explicitly mandating that children with disabilities have the same opportunity for education as children without them. Just like laws that prohibit discrimination on the basis of race, sex, and religion, the ADA is supposed to guarantee that people with disabilities have the same opportunities as everyone else. But just like other civil-rights laws, legislation has not achieved equity, and activists continue the fight.

Nicki Vander Meulen became a disability-rights advocate at age eight in 1986, fighting to attend the local public school in Walworth County, Wisconsin, instead of a school for kids with disabilities. Though she ultimately fought her way into the system, ableism presented an added set of hurdles throughout her public education, hurdles that still exist for children today. In elementary, middle, and high school, peers and authorities picked on Vander Meulen and questioned whether she belonged. In law school at UW-Madison, classmates made derogatory comments and filed complaints about her use of a note-taker. She continues to deal with ableism as a criminal-defense attorney and member of the MMSD Board of Education.

Justice is always about reaching for an ideal, and with school, the ideal is for kids with disabilities to study the same curriculum alongside their peers in the classroom. Decades of research suggest that when students with disabilities are included in a classroom setting designed for all children, they develop stronger math, literacy, communication, and social skills and that it's ultimately good for all kids. But segregation of children in public schools is still widespread.

"Although kids with disabilities are spending more and more time in general classrooms, in the United States, 'special' education still often means 'separate,'" writes Julie Kim, the parent of a daughter with intellectual and physical disabilities, in *The Atlantic* in March 2023. In 2020, fewer than 7 out of 10 students in the US served under the Individuals with Disabilities Education Act spent 80% or more of their time in general classes. Thirty percent spent significant time in segregated classrooms. In the same year, students with disabilities were more than twice as likely as those without disabilities to drop out of high school. "[S]eparate 'special' schools (or siloed classrooms within schools) can sometimes resort to a focus on 'life skills' instead of curriculum-based goals," writes Kim. "Research has indicated that for students with disabilities, an inclusive education can have positive long-term effects on almost every aspect of their lives, including their likelihood of enrolling in college and graduating, finding employment, and forming long-term relationships."

Progressive parents must grasp the truth about disabilities, and the truth about what's at stake. As with other hierarchical power structures, several ableist assumptions perpetuate injustice. The prevailing medical model of disability posits that disability is chiefly a medical issue and that mitigating associated problems is about fixing the individual.

There's been a growing push by activists since the 1960s and 1970s to frame disabilities not as individual deficits but a construct grounded in social inequity. It's a view I take to heart. In 1983, the late Mike Oliver, the first professor of disability studies in the world, who became a wheelchair user after an accident two decades earlier, coined the phrase *social model of disability* to reflect that systemic barriers, social exclusion, and discrimination prevent people with disabilities from participation in a full life according to their values and desires. While some people with disabilities do have medical and social requirements to maximize what they can do, people living with disabilities can also be healthy and are also "normal."

This ideology underlies *universal design*, a term first coined by the architect Ronald L. Mace to describe built environments that can be used by all people to the greatest extent possible. Commonly cited examples of universal design include sidewalk ramps, automatic doors, elevators, nonslip flooring, and wide sidewalks and hallways. Without limiting our environments to what we're used to, entire neighborhoods or cities could be safe and accessible for all people to navigate. In this view of universal design, all people, including our children, could live their most expansive lives. Since the emergence of the social model of disability, however, some disability activists and scholars have warned against painting a too-rosy picture of universal design. The sole focus on the functionality of built environment may not go far enough to challenge ableism. "Critical disability theorists emphasize instead that the design of 'habitable worlds' must involve treating disability itself as a valuable way of being in the world, one that societies must work to accept and preserve rather than cure or rehabilitate," writes Aimi Hamraie, PhD, a disability-justice organizer and director of the Critical Design Lab at Vanderbilt University in a 2016 article. A truly habitable world would "offer more inclusive ideological assumptions about disability, and not simply more accessible structures." Centering the politicized and technical perspectives of disabled designers is crucial to ensure that environments work for people across the spectrum of needs and abilities. Think of what, or who, might be stopping us from creating something like it on a large scale.

Another flawed assumption, based on stereotypes, is that people's disabilities are obvious based on observable characteristics. In reality, many people of all ages, including children, have what's known as *invisible* or *hidden disabilities*, or physical or mental conditions that are not outwardly apparent and that can limit or challenge someone's cognition, movements, or activities. Some people use assistive devices like wheelchairs or canes only part of the time, when needed. Together, misguided assumptions have cemented narrow and ultimately harmful views of disabled people. Children without an obvious disability may be deemed lazy or incapable when they're really struggling with instruction that isn't suited to them. Those with obvious disabilities have been assumed to be less capable than they are, leading to discrimination and stifled opportunities.

The concept of neurodiversity, which represents the broad spectrum of human neurobiology and the many variations in how people experience and interact with the world around them, first emerged in the late 1990s in opposition to the prevailing view that neurodevelopmental disorders are fundamentally pathological. *Neurodiversity* is not a medical term but an umbrella term for differences in the way people's brains work. Since arising from the autism-rights movement decades ago, some concepts of neurodivergence have expanded to include other conditions like ADHD, bipolar disorder, Tourette's syndrome, dyslexia, sensory-processing disorders, and others. Researchers have increasingly adopted the concept in the 2020s with some calling for a shift toward the neurodiversity paradigm to inform scientific studies.

With neurodiversity, which has always been a part of humanity, comes differences in behaviors, mannerisms, communication styles, and perceptions of decorum. In other words, some people act in ways that the majority would deem unconventional. But there isn't actually anything abnormal about behaviors like humming, using tools to manage sensory input, avoiding eye contact, or moving around when one might be expected to sit still. Stimming, or voluntary or involuntary, repetitive, self-stimulatory behavior, like hand-flapping, rocking back and forth, and vocalizing, is normal. Disability-rights activists say that forcing children to mask these behaviors violates their bodily autonomy and freedom to be themselves.

Tiffany Green says that the popularity of the idea that examining our own personal biases is the key to dismantling inequity "ignores that we have these huge power hierarchies and differentials that are reified in all of our institutions." She's not just talking about racism. It also applies to ableism. Systems uphold inequity, and individuals with the power and will to act must do so to change them. "Let's say I want to do implicit-bias training on disability," Green asks hypothetically. "Well, that's cool, but has it changed the fact that buildings aren't accessible?"

Equity means making accommodations to ensure that everyone can thrive and be truly free to make their way throughout the world. Too many establishments have chosen to deprioritize the disabled, acting as if they don't exist, while children have been and are living on the sidelines.

When it came to the COVID-19 pandemic, our systems failed the most vulnerable—people with what doctors call comorbidities or existing medical conditions. "The overwhelming number of deaths, over 75%, occurred in people who had at least 4 comorbidities," said Rochelle Walensky, director of the Centers for Disease Control and Prevention, on a January 7, 2022, segment of *Good Morning America*. She continued, "so really these are people who were unwell to begin with," which she called "really encouraging news in the context of Omicron."

"People heard that only disabled and elderly people would die, and they said, 'Oh, pfft, well, we'll be fine then, right? We'll be okay,'" said Imani Barbarin about the early days of the pandemic.

Changing the world may very well depend on deconstructing the pressure we feel as individual parents. We've all heard the vaguely sciencey-sounding notions that individual failures to live up to ideals around natural birth, exclusive breastfeeding, cooking all-natural meals from scratch, and providing the most stimulating activities can mess up your child for life. **While individual parenting actions have their place, the outsized focus on them can distract from holding systems accountable, ultimately maintaining injustice.** For centuries, wherever capitalism undermined communal childrearing support, individual responsibility has fallen primarily to mothers. Though this unequal pressure is dehumanizing and rests on flawed scientific assumptions, we've been conditioned to think it's totally normal. Ableism infuses this view.

Consider screen time. Parents are told to avoid allowing it

or to minimize it—and we're conditioned to feel guilty about the time our kids do spend with screens. Claim after claim that screen time is rotting kids' brains and creating zoned-out generations lacking connection to nature and family has led to a fear of mobile devices and apps. Studies on associations between screen time and everything from obesity to ADHD have been widely reported in recent decades. The best parents are supposed to spend their time, energy, and income providing stimulating, wholesome activities devoid of screens. Those who fail are supposed to be ashamed. But the truth is a lot less cut-and-dried, and the problem isn't the sheer amount of time spent on screens. The specter of screen time is a feminist issue in large part because it's used as a club to enforce the idealized version of motherhood, which in turn reinforces the notion that a good mother spends a bulk of her bandwidth providing wholesome and low-tech activities for her children. As technology writer and researcher Alexandra Samuel put it in the magazine *JSTOR Daily* on Mother's Day 2016, "When we fret about excess screen time as bad parenting" or "relying on an electronic babysitter" as a "shirking" of duties, "we're really worrying that mothers are putting their own needs alongside, or even ahead of, their kids' needs." This is a worry that "rears its head any time someone comes up with a technology that makes mothers' lives easier."

Among other specters that parents are supposed to take concerted individual action to avoid is their children becoming overweight or obese, and screen time is seen as a major cause of this dreaded outcome. Headlines about the "alarming" link between screen time and pediatric obesity suggest that it's wreaking havoc on waistlines and lives. A doctor writing in *Physician's Weekly* in January of 2022 noted that this association between weight gain and screen time "is due in part to increased sedentary behavior," but it is also associated with "mindless eating behaviors and intake of sugar-sweetened beverages." Again, this sounds benign, scientific, and clinical on its surface—I once would have found it completely acceptable—but to suggest that children of higher weights have uniquely "mindless" behaviors is fatphobic. The assumptions behind much of this research, including that being fat is a child's fault, and that fat is inherently a bad thing, needs to be wiped out of medicine and society for the well-being of all kids. Researchers, clinicians, parents, and activists are increasingly saying that fat is actually far less harmful to children than our aversion to it.

The prevailing message for parents is that it's up to us to do whatever we can to make sure our kids' weight stays under control. This has led to fatphobia, which some call *fatmisia*, directed at children. But it's not really screen time and bad individual choices causing fatness, and it's not actually fatness itself causing harm (note that some activists have reclaimed *fat* as a neutral-to-positive, and not negative, descriptor). Indeed, it's usually a red flag whenever something as varied as screen time is painted with a broad brush and deemed universally bad—Wikipedia and PBS Kids are nothing like internet bullying and unrealistic beauty standards. Yes, we know that social media can cause real harm. But in a world in which loneliness also causes real harm, the human connection that devices can enable is remarkable, though there is a long way to go to make screen time inclusive and more intuitive.

Fatphobia leads to the bulk of these bad outcomes, not fatness itself. We've been told that scaring and shaming children into a normal weight is necessary and worth it to keep them healthy. But the pressure on kids to strive to be thin is unacceptable. Spanking was normal decades ago and is no longer accepted because we know that it's harmful. Fat shaming, along with body shaming of all kinds, is going the same way.

The idea that too much body fat is a moral failure and causes an array of health problems, lack of success, and unhappiness is not only bigoted, it's also not accurate. Doctors, parents, and policymakers have internalized the misguided view that someone's weight is their own doing, and that myth seeps into all public spaces. Underlying the science of human weight is the spurious, essentialist idea that there is such a thing as a normal, healthy weight. While the term *body mass index* was first coined in 1972, the concept has been around for nearly 200 years. A Belgian mathematician by the name of Adolphe Quetelet devised the index in the mid-1800s as part of his study of *l'homme moyen*, or the average man, which looked at a slew of traits. To Quetelet, the human features of the model average man represented the ideal. Then called Quetelet's Index, he based the concept of BMI solely on the measurements of small groups of Western Europeans. By the turn of the next century, the traits studied in *l'homme moyen* would be used as a scientific justification for eugenics, including the sterilization of disabled people, autistic people, people experiencing poverty, and non-Europeans. Quetelet never intended BMI to be an individual indicator of health or well-being.

Throughout much of human history, with its famines and plagues, fatness has been seen as a sign of prosperity, power, health, and wealth in many cultures, separating those who live in relative leisure from those who toil and scrounge. But that view started shifting two hundred years ago. By the nineteenth century, articles in magazines warning middle-class and upper-class white women that they needed to watch what they ate were common, "and they were unapologetic in stating that this was the proper form for Anglo-Saxon Protestant women," Sabrina Strings, PhD, an assistant professor of sociology at the University of California, Irvine, says in a 2020 *NPR* interview. When researching her 2019 book, *Fearing the Black Body: The Racial Origins of Fat Phobia*, she found that these magazines relied on flawed European colonizer logic. They figured "that Africans are sensuous. They love sex, and they love food" and therefore "they tend to be too fat." By contrast, Europeans told themselves that they "have rational self-control," which made them "the premier race of the world," she explains.

In reality, weight is simply not a great proxy for well-being. The insurance industry, which isn't known for its integrity, is what transformed the concept of BMI into one that's applied to individuals as an indicator of health. In the early twentieth century, life insurance companies created tables of height and weight to calculate what to charge policyholders. Largely arbitrarily, physicians began to adopt these measures, and by 1985, the National Institutes of Health had revised their definition of *obesity* to be tied to individual patients' BMIs.

The prevailing fear of fat gained momentum in the late 1990s when there was a concerted push to convince Americans that there was an unprecedented *obesity epidemic*. As the story goes, despite concerted efforts, obesity rates have risen alarmingly in recent decades. The media consistently reinforces that obesity is a matter of personal responsibility, but the idea that weight is about willpower is a systemic, fatal application of that old fundamental attribution error. What's glossed over in our collective memory is that, in 1998, the National Institutes of Health substantially lowered the threshold to be considered *overweight* and *obese*. As CNN reported in its health section, "Millions of Americans became 'fat' Wednesday—even if they didn't gain a pound." Charts depicting startling spikes in the portion of Americans, children included, who were overweight or obese were everywhere without reference to the changes in the definitions of those words. This was grossly misleading, revved resentment of fat individuals, and added another layer of justification for medical mistreatment. Without consideration of the conditions that influence body fat, like discrimination, stress, lack of sleep, green spaces, and access to food, systemic fatphobia made children and their mothers a main target of the war against obesity. But individual behaviors that are widely assumed to cause fatness, like screen time, lack of willpower, or laziness, have never been the real problem.

Unvarnished history largely shows that, when not subjected to famine, humans have naturally always come in a spectrum of shapes and sizes. There have always been fat people whom we would consider healthy by most measures and thin folks with health problems. More useful indicators include lean muscle mass, which is good for the body, and measures of metabolic health including blood sugar, blood pressure, cholesterol, and triglyceride levels.

Once the concept of the ideal weight took hold, in addition to the personal-responsibility narrative, it wasn't long before the racist idea that fatness is a genetic trait that is statistically more prevalent in certain ethnicities, especially Black girls and women, gained traction. Activists have been fighting this notion since its inception, and it's no different in the 2020s. Jennifer Tsai is among that throng of heroes. "We write to call attention to the authors' problematic assumptions about race, which were particularly concerning to see in an influential publication," she and her coauthors say in an August 2020 letter to the editor of the *Journal of Internal Medicine*.

The problematic paper, published on April 29, 2020, is a literature review that seeks to determine genetic variables that cause higher rates of obesity in African-American women based on the flawed assumption that race is genetic. Lead author Barbara Gower, PhD, is a professor in the Department of Nutrition Sciences Division of Physiology and Metabolism at the University of Alabama at Birmingham. Her work funded by the US NIH at this public-research university takes as its basis that there is a physiological and genetic reason for the observed higher rate of obesity in African-American women compared to Caucasian or European-American women. In other words, the fallacious assumption of the genetic segregation of so-called races is built into their research. One would be justified in calling it hateful and pseudoscientific. Nonetheless, whiteness deftly cloaks racism in the trappings of legitimate inquiry.

The rebuttal by Tsai et al. to Gower and Fowler goes on to explain that the researchers' premise in their May 2020 review paper on "the role of physiology" in obesity among "African-Americans"—the assumption of racial essentialism, or the notion that there are consistent genomic, innate differences between so-called races—is woefully flawed. Gower and Fowler's review article presumes that Black women are inherently "obesity-prone" and uses computational analyses of observational data from previous studies to propose a genetic explanation for the disparity. Without genetic evidence to support their hypothesis, the authors surmise that Black women's bodies convert calories to more fat than white women's bodies. They didn't actually find a genetic reason for the disparity because there isn't one. Rather, they used their paper to propose a hypothesis that there must be one and to argue that their proposed genetic reason is worth further investigation.

"This inference is unacceptable," write Tsai and her coauthors in their rebuttal. "It produces illegitimate science that reifies racial determinism and obfuscates the contribution of structural racism to racial health inequalities." The rebuttal by Tsai and her peers was one of a few that called out the racism inherent in Gower's research, which continues to receive NIH funding.

Gower and Fowler responded to Tsai and colleagues in a follow-up letter published in the same journal, writing, "We believe that refraining from reporting scientific findings because of fear of political discomfort (in this case racism) is a violation to scientific integrity."

Acting like obesity occurs in genetically and morally faulty individuals has helped institutions continue to do nothing about the conditions that harm children of all shapes and sizes. Fatphobia is among the most socially accepted form of bigotry, and it starts affecting children before kindergarten. Until recently, the harms of weight stigma itself have not received the same attention as ostensible health-related outcomes of fatness like heart disease and diabetes. Scientists are only starting to figure out how exactly stigma affects children's bodies and minds. There seems to be a negative feedback loop: stigma, in the form of bullying from peers, comments and restrictions in the home, or discrimination by educators, can contribute to reduced participation in activities, lower self-esteem, depression and anxiety, unhealthy eating behaviors that can cause eating disorders and changes to metabolic health, and even, ironically, weight gain. The ubiquitous belief—among doctors, parents, educators, researchers, and everyone, really—is that children and adults of higher weights are lazy or lack willpower. In reality, someone's body weight is the result of complex interactions among several physiological, biological, psychological, social, and environmental factors. These include genetics, epigenetics, hormones, stress, food insecurity, food policies, and school, home, and neighborhood environments.

Fatphobia and medical obsession with BMI has failed generations of children by justifying prejudice and discrimination, which contribute to poor health outcomes. It will continue to do so until people force systems to dismantle it. Though too many weight-loss interventions that target kids rely on shame, fear, and judgment, fatphobic BMI-centric pressure doesn't motivate weight loss. Large studies of interventions designed to get people to a specific BMI or supposedly ideal goal weight have shown that they don't work very well. Diet, exercise, and/or medication lead to no more than 10% body-weight loss on average, and for the most part, ending the intervention leads to weight regain.

Indeed, for parents who grew up in the age of ultrathin supermodels, whose ideal of beauty came paired with an ideal of personal discipline, it's mind-boggling to learn that weight is not about willpower and fatness doesn't dictate well-being. It's easier for systems to blame our kids' health problems on fatness and screen time. Generalizations about body size and health behaviors harm people of all sizes, not just those who are visibly bigger. Evidence suggests that contrary to the prevailing wisdom, losing weight isn't particularly helpful in people with higher BMIs who are otherwise healthy. Research increasingly suggests that a good chunk of fat people are healthy by several measures, while those with a so-called healthy weight can have heart disease, diabetes, high cholesterol, and eating disorders. Remember that, on the whole, kids are supposed to gain weight throughout childhood.

As the fight for change continues, parenting with feminism requires changing the way we think and talk about race and gender, letting go of common ableist thinking, and teaching our children to do the same. Modeling disability inclusion and antiableism in our own backyards is key, and again, part of that is inclusive language. Think of words like *stupid, dumb, crazy,* or *lame.* People throw them around a lot to describe either harmful or misguided actions and views, like shitty business practices, political missteps, everyday mistakes, or your favorite fast-food joint's broken soft-serve machine, to name a sliver of examples. These ableist words are so ubiquitous that they don't seem out of place at all. At first, it was hard for me to stop using them, but, though I do slip up at times and fall back on them, especially when I'm tired or drained, I continue to correct myself and stay committed because my kids are watching. When I do hear my children use these words uncritically, I point out the inherent ableism and ask them to think of a more accurate descriptor for their needs. I try to do the same when I encounter these words among the adults in my circles. I ask questions like *Is it really stupid to drop the ball, or is it a lack of foresight? Is it really crazy to suggest that a legitimate election was stolen, or is it fascist? Is it really dumb to have to stand in line for way too long because the store is understaffed, or is it capitalistic greed?*

When possible, fighting ableism in our own backyards can be as simple as thinking about others. Even among well-meaning people, it can be "hard for them to think outside their own experience," says Alexis Record, a writer, activist, and parent of two special-needs children based in San Diego, California. Lack of inclusion has had an undeniable impact on their lives as it does on millions of kids. When they were young, her kids' "entire class would be invited" to a party, "we would show up and couldn't physically get into the front door." This has led to them attending fewer birthday parties. If you're hosting a gathering, instead of waiting until the day of, ask about what kids need to participate in an event or activity ahead of time. Their caregivers will almost always be glad you asked, Record says.

It's taken some work, but I've also learned to worry less about screen time and weight and more about teaching our children to take care of themselves and each other. Anastasia Bodnar often shares tips, including that "media can enhance daily life" when used appropriately. She encourages parents to "do your homework on educational apps," because while many apps are labeled *educational*, "little research has demonstrated their quality." When in doubt about how to navigate screen time, there are resources like the ones at Commonsense Media, a nonprofit organization that works to make technology safer, healthier, and more equitable for kids everywhere and provides resources for families to help children safely get the most out of screens and practice good digital citizenship (while always staying vigilant).

Guidelines for caregivers on media use for children from the American Academy of Pediatrics explain that "[t]here are risks and benefits that come with media use, and the key is to develop habits that help your family strike a healthy balance."

"You can decide what media use is best for your family. Remember, all children and teens need adequate sleep (eight to twelve hours, depending on age), physical activity (one hour), and time away from media." They also point out that the approach isn't one-size-fits-all. Children have highly personalized media use experiences, so "parents must develop personalized media use plans for their children." Consider each child's age, health, personality, interests, and developmental stage, and consult a pediatrician with questions.

In May of 2023, the American Psychological Association released a health advisory on social-media use in adolescence. It points out that using social media "is not inherently beneficial or harmful" to youth. "Adolescents' lives online both reflect and impact their offline lives." In most cases the effects of social media depend largely on personal characteristics and circumstances. Social-media use "should be based on each adolescent's level of maturity (e.g., self-regulation skills, intellectual development, comprehension of risks) and home environment."

Celebrating all bodies while changing systems and promoting well-being—not thinness—is what will really protect our children from the bad things that we want to prevent and promote the outcomes we want to encourage. Some of our parents pressured us about our weight, and I know that we can break this generational trauma. They thought that by pushing us to be thin, they were pushing us toward success. Now we know that this couldn't have been more wrong. Our children's bodies are beautiful, powerful vessels of precious life, and we need to make sure they know it. Rather than urging individual children who are categorized as *overweight* or *obese* to lose weight, systemic change that creates the healthiest environments for all kids, and fosters love for their bodies, is the way forward. In making this change, we need to dismantle the hate we progressive parents have internalized about our own bodies starting in childhood or adolescence and model love for ourselves because our children are watching. There are no inherently good foods or bad foods. All foods can be good in the right context and appropriate proportions and amounts for each person. Striving to consume the nutrients we need while enjoying them—and doing anything in our power to ensure that everyone else can, too—is the goal. The Eurocentric idea that the Mediterranean diet is healthier than others is simply untrue. All of the world's cuisines can be nutritious and healthy.

Physical activity isn't a duty tied to achieving or maintaining a so-called normal weight. It is about doing what makes us feel good and striving to reach the physical goals we have for ourselves, like getting out of bed, spiking a volleyball, lifting heavier things, being present with loved ones, climbing higher, breathing easier, building a snowman, kneading bread, turning the pages of a book, dancing, throwing dice, feeling good, and anything in between and beyond.

Modeling inclusivity is an ongoing task, and it doesn't require perfection, only concerted effort. By and large, one of the most revolutionary feminist urges is also one of the most fundamental ways to protect our children—the urge to build up their self-love and love for others.

6

a clean life

There's an old chemistry parody warning that goes something like this: the ubiquitous chemical Dihydrogen Monoxide (DHMO) causes widespread harm. Also known as hydric acid, this colorless, odorless, tasteless compound kills thousands of people every year, and its dangers are underrecognized. It's used as an industrial solvent, in the application of pesticides, and as an additive in processed foods. Exposure to its solid form can cause tissue damage and bruises, and inhalation can result in brain damage and death, including in children and even babies. It has been found in the blood of all people with cancer, diabetes, and autoimmune disease. Due to widespread lobbying for the industrial use of this compound, campaigns to ban DHMO have failed. The warning often comes paired with a poll asking whether the information warrants banning this dangerous chemical. The answer is often *yes*.

The spoof here is that Dihydrogen Monoxide is an unfamiliar name for *water*, the molecule that consists of two hydrogen atoms and an oxygen atom, or H2O. Since the 1980s, a faction of those who want to demonstrate the absurdity of *chemophobia*—or fear of chemicals—have used DHMO scare tactics to expose gullible belief in unsubstantiated fear-mongering. It's a manifestation of chemists' frustration with what they see as the public's lack of science literacy around chemistry and their dismay at the resulting proliferation of products and trends that claim to be "chemical-free" or "free from" so-called toxic chemicals. Academia and industry groups lament perceived widespread chemophobia. Even the journal *Nature Chemistry* joined the show of frustration, publishing a parody paper in 2014 detailing a comprehensive list of chemical-free consumer products. It was an introduction followed by two blank pages, meant to serve as a humorous visual demonstration. The world's chemists love to catch people in these jokes to exhibit that all matter is made of chemicals. They are attempting to convey the basic tenet of toxicology that the dose makes the poison. Anything can be harmful when taken in harmful concentrations.

But there's evidence to suggest that people aren't as gullible about chemicals as frustrated chemists assume. To study whether members of the lay public are really clueless enough to believe that all chemicals are bad, in 2015, the Royal Society of Chemistry, a British professional association, conducted a survey on attitudes about chemistry in the UK. Of those polled, 60% agreed that "everything is made of chemicals," and 70% agreed that "everything, including water and oxygen, can be toxic at a certain dose." Writing of his team's results, Prof. Mark Lorch, chemist and science communicator, admitted that his field has largely underestimated chemical literacy. "What is particularly telling about the RSC's findings is not that the public doesn't understand chemists, but that chemists don't understand the public." As he put it, people are "'quite capable of holding two meanings of 'chemical' in their mind." I find it refreshing when scientists can admit they were coming from a haughty place, but I don't think Lorch's humility is common among scientists.

Molecules are all around us. What we want to know is which chemicals are problematic, whether they're harmful to children or the planet, and whether they're tied to predatory, exploitative, or unethical practices. The discourse around a so-called clean life is about avoiding the chemicals that we're told are toxic, especially when they're synthetic, and embracing the more wholesome, wellness-promoting, natural ones. Consider food and agriculture. Food-industry players with different professed values aim to land customers with dovetailing worldviews. Sometimes, these players themselves aim to harness or pervade those worldviews in their customer base, influencing food choices and eating trends. *Clean eating* and related ideologies raise the question of what, exactly, *clean* food is. Many of us define it for ourselves or figure that clean eating must be a good thing, and that it makes sense for parents to avoid feeding children harmful chemicals. But the meaning of *clean* isn't as clear as one would imagine. It depends in large part on who you ask. The USDA and Health and Human Services provide Dietary Guidelines for Americans (DGA), which include advice on meeting nutrient needs, promoting health, and preventing disease. Nowhere in the 2020–2025 DGA is *clean eating* mentioned at all with regard to problematic chemicals. The word *clean* does appear in the context of safe food-handling practices to prevent foodborne illness from pathogens, like hand-washing and keeping food-prep surfaces clean, and cooking foods to safe internal temperatures. The guidelines also use the word *clean* to refer to the safe handling of infant formula and human milk. Similar to the DGA, the FDA's idea of clean eating is to promote food safety. The Academy of Nutrition and Dietetics, a trade association that represents over a hundred thousand credentialed nutrition and dietetics practitioners, doesn't take a stance on clean eating, either.

None of this is to say that parents should dismiss *clean* living outright. There are chemicals in our communities and homes that can harm our children. **The problem is that some of the chemicals we're told to worry about are far more harmful than others. We're faced with a massive mix of credible and spurious information, a lot of which appears legitimate on the surface.** In the parenting realm, different stakeholders focus on what they sometimes call *chemicals of concern* in food, household products, personal-care products, medicine, and the environment. Some of the more common fears over specific chemicals are unfounded at best and downright misleading at worst, distracting us from, well, everything we should actually worry about. Do the lists of chemicals we're supposed to avoid enable us to protect our children and help them thrive?

Consider MSG, that flavoring that we often associate with Chinese food. Since 2017, Panera has been one food brand and manufacturer leading the clean-eating charge with its *100% Clean* slogan and *Food as It Should Be* promise. In pursuit of fulfilling its clean pledge, the company eliminated a so-called no-no list of artificial preservatives, sweeteners, flavors, and colors from its restaurant menu and grocery items, including MSG. As of this writing, there are a couple of products with *No MSG* labels in my family's kitchen, including a package of frozen breakfast sausages.

Fellow SciParent Layla Katiraee recalls avoiding MSG during her time in China while she was pregnant, believing that it would be better not to ingest it. I remember regularly asking for no MSG at my favorite local Chinese take-out place years ago. MSG aversion is common, with many believing that it causes headaches, dizziness, or palpitations—a set of symptoms sometimes known as "Chinese restaurant syndrome." While we've been led to believe that it is an inherently nefarious and unnatural additive that the big food industry uses to addict children to junk, MSG is about as artificial as granulated sugar. It's practically as natural as life on Earth. And as much as we associate

MSG with Chinese food, there isn't anything inherently Asian about it. Scholars have noted that Americans rejected MSG in large part because of negative feelings about Chinese people in the 1960s and '70s. In recent years, MSG aversion has been viewed through the lens of the xenophobia and racism that fueled it, and the role that these views played in the trajectory of science.

MSG stands for *monosodium glutamate*, the sodium salt of glutamate, which is an amino acid that the human body can synthesize, and that we also get from our food. It breaks down into glutamate and salt when ingested, and is the purest form of umami which, along with sweet, sour, bitter, and salty, is one of the five basic tastes that our tongues are thought to perceive. Glutamate is an important building block for proteins, and it also helps nerve cells send signals throughout the body. Humans have umami-specific receptors on our tongues and in our stomachs, and these receptors whet our cravings for foods that contain it, like tomatoes, mushrooms, cheese, and, for babies, human milk and infant formula. Umami-rich foods have been staples in human diets for as far back as historians look. Cultures have been concentrating available, naturally occurring glutamate by sun-drying tomatoes, curing meat, and fermenting vegetables for centuries, long before we knew what amino acids were.

Humanity came upon pure MSG in 1908, when Prof. Kikunae Ikeda, a Japanese chemist, realized that the kombu seaweed in his soup imparted a flavor that wasn't one of the four established tastes. He isolated the crystalline salt of glutamate from kelp and made culinary history. He called the MSG crystals *Ajinomoto*, a Japanese word meaning *the essence of taste*, and developed a process to mass-produce it. Back then, it was isolated from seaweed and then crystallized with salt during the drying process, and today it's usually produced using fermented sugarcane, sugar beets, or corn. In Asia, it was branded a staple and quickly became ubiquitous in kitchens across Japan and China.

I've come to think of it this way: adding MSG to food is about as natural as adding regular table salt or sugar. All of these substances occur in nature and are present in living organisms, and humans have learned to concentrate and isolate them for various uses. The glutamate in MSG is chemically identical to the glutamate present in animal and plant proteins, just like table sugar is chemically identical to the sucrose that occurs naturally in plants.

For those who grew up seeing their grandparents sprinkle MSG into saucepans from a jar occupying a central place in the kitchen, the decades-long aversion to it has stung. That aversion to the seasoning has roots in a 1968 letter to the editor published in the *New England Journal of Medicine* describing the author's and his friends' so-called Chinese restaurant syndrome after eating Chinese food, including symptoms like heart palpitations, generalized weakness, and radiating numbness. The idea took hold, spurring years of biased research based on the flawed assumption that the syndrome is a real thing that also includes symptoms like headaches and nausea, and that MSG causes it.

Based on this assumption, subsequent animal studies seemingly confirmed that MSG caused the alleged syndrome, but these studies often consisted of injecting superconcentrated doses of MSG directly into creatures' abdomens, which is not exactly a scientific approach to studying the effects of a substance that we ingest at much lower doses. Over the last thirty years, a number of double-blinded, placebo-controlled studies, including studies of subjects with reported sensitivity to MSG, have failed to find a reproducible response to eating it in food. But all of that hasn't stopped aversion to MSG. There's no shortage of *Yelp* reviews complaining about headaches and palpitations after consuming stir-fry and egg rolls, and a slew of restaurants that trot out MSG-free offerings. Like the sausages with the *No MSG* claim in our freezer that our kids eat often, which most definitely contain glutamate, many of these claims are misleading.

Like so many other parenting questions that involve science, the case of MSG and so-called Chinese restaurant syndrome shows that claims about chemicals being harmful aren't always true. **So how do you know which chemicals to worry about? Fortunately, a few concepts surrounding chemicals can help us navigate this terrain.**

Alison Bernstein, who knows the fear and confusion around chemicals all too well, has had a transformation in her views as a parent and has used what she's learned to help others. Not even a decade ago, she recounts that grocery shopping was an "anxiety-filled experience." In 2009, when her daughter was one, she joined a lab with a focus on neurotoxicology research at the Emory University Rollins School of Public Health for her first postdoctoral position. She was certain that she would gain the knowledge she'd need to avoid all toxicants for her kids and guarantee them a 100% risk-free life. Instead, she learned that her own preconceived ideas about risk were not evidence-based. She points out that people with agendas often use confusion around risk-related concepts to manipulate parents. Evidence strongly suggests that humans are innately bad at assessing risk. "Risks are not always intuitive, and our cognitive shortcuts can lead us astray," write Bernstein and coauthor Iida Ruishalme in a 2018 blog series putting risk-related concepts into perspective for parents. This can "complicate our ability to make informed decisions about" vaccines, the food we eat and feed our children, and so much more.

Think about the chemicals used in farming. In 2015, the Coop chain of grocery stores, known as a pioneer for organic food in Sweden, with hundreds of locations in the country, partnered with the Swedish Environmental Research Institute to conduct an experiment on two parents and their three adorable blond kids for three weeks. The family, which ate a conventional, nonorganic diet to keep food costs down, switched to organic for two weeks, giving daily urine samples.

The results were presented in a video called "The Organic Effect," which went viral globally. The Swedish video with English voiceover and subtitles claimed that before switching to organic, the family's urine contained agricultural chemicals. "We're eating pesticides," says one of the children.

"Disgusting," replies the mother.

According to charts presented in the video, after eating an all-organic diet for two weeks, the chemicals were no longer there. "Now, almost all the pesticides have disappeared."

With tens of millions of views across social-media platforms and news coverage worldwide, the "Organic Effect" video brought the concern over pesticides in our children's bodies to the forefront. "Family eats organic for just two weeks, removes nearly all pesticides from body," read a headline from the *Sydney Morning Herald* following the video's release.

The narrative has its draws. A family of five goes from pesticide-ridden to immaculate urine in just two weeks. "There were a whole number of chemicals removed from my kids' bodies, and I don't want them back," explained the concerned mom in the video. The message is that our children's health is worth the price premium for organic, which is compelling on its surface, but the video doesn't tell the whole story. Remember that when industries eliminate the use of a specific substance, they almost always switch to using something else instead to perform the same or similar function. By and large, farmers use chemicals to grow crops in the most profitable way, including pesticides, and organic farming is no different.

Even though organic farming on a large scale uses chemicals, it's no surprise that people think organic farming is chemical-free. In a post for her "Bad Chart Thursday" series, Melanie Mallon—who was part of the crew at *Skepchick* sibling site *Grounded Parents* where SciParent Jenny Splitter and I both started blogging—delved into what she calls "organic cherry-picking." Mallon explains that the poorly designed experiment showed exactly what we'd expect when dropping convention-ally grown food: the level of pesticides used in conventional farming detected in the family's urine went down drastically. Evidence suggests that organic-market growth is fueled in part by misleading information from certain groups that denigrate conventionally grown food, including wordplay that implies or outright asserts that organic farming doesn't use pesticides or is better for health. This manipulation works because organic farming gives off an impression of being closer to nature, and anything natural seems more gentle and health-promoting. But organic labels don't tell us whether foods were produced on smaller farms or with good working conditions or more hu-mane and environmentally friendly farming practices. The only thing an organic label tells us is that a product was sourced from organic-certified facilities.

Different countries have different regulatory schemes for their organic producers. In the United States, the National Organic Program is the regulatory body that oversees which chemicals and other practices are allowed and prohibited for seed suppliers, farmers, food processors, retailers, restaurants, and textile man-ufacturers that use an *organic* seal or label. All governing agen-cies that oversee organic certification around the world allow agricultural chemicals, including pesticides.

The "Organic Effect" video omitted the fact that organic farming does use pesticides, albeit different than the ones used in conventional agriculture. Coop's experiment didn't test for pesticides used in organic production. Even though the pesti-cides approved for use in organic farming tend to be naturally derived, whether a substance is synthetic or natural in origin has no bearing on its toxicity in and of itself. Along with brush-ing over the existence of pesticides used in organic farming, the video failed to mention that the levels of chemicals detected in the experiment pose no known risk to children. The video's narrative did its job, as millions liked and shared it.

"[T]his experiment could easily be conducted by testing only for organic pesticide levels and we would see an empty or near-empty 'Before Organic' chart followed by an 'After Organic' chart showing pesticide levels," wrote Mallon. "Could we then conclude that organic is poisoning our children? Probably not any more than this advertisement can make the opposite claim. That we have chemicals in our body tells us nothing about whether those chemicals in those amounts are harmful."

The following year, the Swedish Crop Protection Association (*Svenskt Växtskydd*) filed a lawsuit against Coop for misleading and inaccurate advertising. The association, which consists of nine separate companies that produce pesticides, argued that the marketing campaign was unethical. In 2017, the court ruled that Coop must cease its misleading claims or face a penalty fine. By then, the video had already made its mark on parents.

With headquarters in Washington, DC, the nonprofit Environmental Working Group (EWG) has been among the most successful US organizations at tapping into chemophobia, focusing on parents, and moms specifically, as a key audience. Its famous annual Dirty Dozen list names the specific conventionally grown fruits and veggies that harbor what they say are alarming pesticide residues that can harm people who eat them, especially children. The organization, its celebrity spokespeople, and its associates urge parents to skip buying conventionally grown fruits and veggies containing the most supposedly toxic residues and opt for organic instead. In 2023, blueberries, spinach, kale, strawberries, grapes, and bell peppers are among the dozen deemed dirty. EWG appears to care about empowering parents, but their messaging effectively confuses folks by suggesting that organic food is imperative for our children's health. The fallacious yet pervasive idea that I should fear feeding my children the perfectly healthy conventionally grown fruit in our kitchen while there are actually harmful chemicals in my community harming children right now is what scares me.

It seems to make sense to think that something should be avoided completely if it has not been proven completely safe. Because humans are hardwired to misperceive risk, and because the thought of something bad happening to our children is so unbearable, leveraging this urge can be profitable. Companies misrepresent the relevant science to create a market for their products based on this instinct.

But it's virtually impossible to prove something completely safe. We know that nothing, not even pure water, is completely safe at all doses and modes of exposure. **Though a no-harm guarantee is appealing, safety is about the likelihood and severity of harm. As much as we yearn for absolute safety, zero risk to our children in any given moment is, as Bernstein often puts it, "an impossible dream."** The question is always a matter of how safe is safe enough. To me, accepting this gray area around safety feels equal parts unsettling and empowering. Yes, we love our children more than life itself, which compels us to act to protect them at all costs. But sometimes, the actions we take to protect them are no more effective than my incessant obsessive-compulsive counting of my newborn's breaths and checking of the stove knobs. No amount of checking and counting could have guaranteed total safety. Meanwhile, I expended energy and forfeited peace to take those actions.

Unpacking a few key risk-related concepts can empower parents. The first is the distinction between *hazard* and *risk*. A hazard is anything with the potential to cause harm, like chemicals in tap water, and risk measures the likelihood of harm from that hazard, like the likelihood of contaminated water causing a specific medical problem. Bernstein stresses that hazards only become risks when there is *exposure*; in other words, risk is largely a measure of the potential for harm + exposure. Families who live in Finland and Iceland have the lowest exposure to harmful chemicals in drinking water. Families who live in parts of the USA with high levels of certain contaminants in drinking water, by contrast, have a much higher risk of associated health effects.

To assess how risky a hazard is and what to do about it, Bernstein often asks parents to think of a graph divided into four quadrants that roughly place hazards into four categories based on the potential for harm and exposure for any hazard. The x-axis represents how many people are exposed to a hazard on a population level, and the y-axis represents the severity of potential harm from that hazard.

Hazards that cause a relatively low severity of harm to relatively few members of the general public, like hot peppers, go in the lower-left quadrant. Certain occupational hazards like climbing cell towers or fighting fires go in the upper-left quadrant because they can cause severe harm like injury or death from falls or burns or lung damage but primarily affect people in specific professions. In the lower-right quadrant, we place hazards that many people are exposed to but pose a relatively low severity of harm, like rhinoviruses, the most common cause of coldlike illnesses. Finally, hazards that have the potential to cause severe consequences to a relatively high number of people, like cigarette smoking, extremely hot weather, and intoxicated drivers, go in the upper-right quadrant, which is where what we would consider the worst hazards go. Though synthetic hazards can seem inherently riskier, whether or not a chemical is naturally derived has no bearing on its healthfulness or toxicity to humans.

Risk often also depends on the type of exposure. Plenty of people regret their decision to eat those hellfire wings or *fuego* chips, but the aftermath is almost never sickening or deadly. Capsaicin poses a different risk to people eating it in food than it does to those exposed to chemical weapons that contain it. But some of the hottest pepper varieties on Earth with the highest capsaicin content have been known to cause nasty effects like burns in the throat and esophagus. And you wouldn't want to eat capsaicin from a tube of topical pain-relief cream containing it as an active ingredient.

Hazards affect different individuals in different ways and can pose different levels of harm depending on exposure, genetics, someone's size, and more. The same hazards can show up in different quadrants when looking at different groups with different exposures and degrees of susceptibility: respiratory viruses, for instance, go much lower and farther to the left for those with no chronic health conditions and farther up and to the right for those who have asthma or are immunocompromized or disabled, among others. Placing hazards into risk quadrants isn't instinctual. Some hazards seem riskier than they are while others that are relatively dangerous don't seem particularly risky. Our understanding of risk evolves as more data comes in. On the whole, the objective for regulatory and public-health agencies, and others tasked with caring for kids, is to minimize risk from various hazards to children, reducing the number of individuals exposed and the severity of the impact. Ideally, policymakers work to protect not just the healthiest and most privileged by and large but those who are the most vulnerable to any hazards.

Today, thanks to an increase in car-seat and seat-belt requirements in the US and other countries, car rides are far less risky for infants and toddlers than they used to be. Meanwhile, when I visit my family in India, I see small children riding on the back seats of motorcycles or in adults' laps, weaving through traffic. In countries without the resources and ability to enact and enforce infant car-seat and seat-belt mandates, the risk of traffic-related injury or death for children remains much higher for far more of the population. And of course, governments don't always act on this objective to push hazards as low and far to the left on these risk quadrants as possible, sometimes erring on the side of political interests, like when Rochelle Walensky implied that letting some groups of people die from COVID was okay.

For parents, it makes sense to grasp exposures as a concept. We don't perceive that our children are exposed to hazards every single moment of their lives. It sounds extreme, but it's true. All foods are choking hazards to people of all ages. Official guidelines to cut grapes into quarters and avoid popcorn and other specific foods until age four have reduced, but not eliminated, the risk of choking in young children. No matter what we do as parents, there are small risks to children all the time, even when they're sleeping peacefully, even in the safest neighborhoods and dwellings. Then when they're awake and out and about? Forget it. Ruminating on all of the hazards around our children is understandable for anxious parents. Accepting that we can't control all of them allows us to focus on what we can control.

We also need to consider the health-promoting exposures for kids, like fresh, clean outdoor air, reading a book, playing in the woods, a good tooth-brushing, a bonding moment with a puppy, laughing with loved ones, the feeling of being seen and accepted, or a bowl of fruit. Every exposure changes us, and exposures are constantly happening, from birth to death. Collectively, all of an individual's exposures in a lifetime, and their complex influence on health, is called the *exposome*. The suffix-*ome* as used in biology refers to a totality of some sort. The genome is the totality of genetic material in the nuclei of an individual's cells. The phenome is the totality of observable traits exhibited by a cell, tissue, organism, or species. Exposures affect the epigenome, those chemical markers over the genome that tells genes when and where to do different things in the body. Exposures also affect someone's microbiome, which is the general term for the entirety of a microbial community, including viruses, bacteria, and fungi, in an individual organism or habitat. Parents hear a lot about the -omes and their impact on kids. **Many influencers claim that their tips, tricks, and products can harness the -omes and their impact on brain health, weight, developmental disorders, and more.** While the microbiome's influence on human health is very real, advice on how to control and shape our microbial community of critters, and products that claim to do so, are not credible. "[T]here is harm in giving false hope to people with all kinds of chronic conditions," microbiologist Elisabeth Bik, formerly a research associate at Stanford School of Medicine, known for her work advocating for scientific integrity, told me in 2016. "Microbiome research is still a very young field, and it is much too early to claim that we know how to use our microbiome to solve chronic heart and gut conditions, autoimmune diseases, and diabetes."

While studies have continued to shed light on the microbiome and data has accumulated, not a whole lot has changed since 2016. "There are almost no examples out there for evidence-based approaches to optimizing one's microbiome," Jonathan Eisen, professor at the Genome Center at the University of California, Davis, tells me in a 2023 email. Though he regularly professes his "love" for microbiome research and his personal belief that we will find "more and more important connections between microbiomes and the health and well-being of plants, animals, other organisms, and ecosystems," Eisen also regularly calls out the widespread "overselling" of the microbiome and what the current body of research tells us. Eisen stresses that, even in 2023, most studies "are still correlative" and "have not shown any actual benefits" that translate to health.

Yes, the epigenome and microbiome have very real influences on our well-being. There's even evidence, largely from animal studies, that trauma changes the epigenome in ways that can be passed from generation to generation. But the vast majority of claims that avoiding this chemical or taking that supplement or switching to a revolutionary diet will heal and optimize the epigenome and microbiome simply don't have the evidence to back them. Everything that we interact with leads to epigenetic changes and impacts the microbes in and on our bodies, and scientists are only beginning to understand the dynamics of these complex interactions. A few of the main evidence-based actions someone can take to optimize their kids' microbiomes include avoiding unnecessary antibiotics, which can throw off the balance of a child's gut microbes, taking a probiotic when you do need to use antibiotics, and practicing food safety and hand hygiene. Living in a neighborhood with safe air and water, having relaxing and fulfilling experiences, getting enough sleep, and eating plenty of fruits and vegetables are protective exposures, and research suggests that they help balance out the negative effects of bad exposures on the epigenome.

As a concept, it's also worth accepting that risk itself is population-based. It doesn't translate neatly to individuals. Bernstein points out that we tend to think in very small sample sizes and not in terms of populations, especially when we're thinking about the well-being of our own families. But epidemiology involves population risks rather than individuals. If something is reported to increase the risk of disease in a population, like an overweight BMI increasing the risk of diabetes, does that mean that this increased risk of developing diabetes applies to any individual child with an overweight BMI? No. Extrapolating a population-level risk to an individual one doesn't work. In other words, you can't look at a fat child and a thin child and assume that the fat one is far more likely to develop diabetes, but we do it anyway. It does children of all sizes a disservice.

In thinking about risk, Bernstein refers to an image of a clear glass jar, in a 2022 paper in *npj Parkinson's Disease*, on how to communicate about risk for Parkinson's. The authors explain that "everyone has a 'Parkinson's jar.'" Environmental factors are represented by small light blue beads, and genetic risk factors are yellow beads. Everyone starts out with yellow beads in their jar for the genetic factors they inherit, some with more than others. Over time, environmental beads also accumulate, and Parkinson's develops once the beads hit a threshold. This jar model roughly works to think of risk for many different conditions, from various forms of cancer to diabetes to autoimmune diseases to chronic pain.

In recent years, scientists have developed methods of chemical detection that can measure smaller and smaller traces of substances. These methods help shed light on complex molecular interactions, enabling improved monitoring and regulation of potentially harmful exposures. But just because we have the ability to detect that some potentially harmful substance is present in tiny amounts doesn't mean that it's harmful in those amounts. As much as we might want to do so, removing all traces of unwanted substances in our environment is another impossible goal, says Bernstein.

Let's consider glyphosate, the key ingredient in Roundup—originally produced by agrichemical giant Monsanto, which Bayer acquired in 2018—and compare and contrast it with a couple of other chemicals. Often used with crops genetically engineered to tolerate it, glyphosate is the most widely used herbicide in the US. As an herbicide, glyphosate blocks the action of an enzyme that enables protein synthesis in living plants. The same pathway doesn't exist in humans, so glyphosate doesn't kill human cells. When applied on fields with crops engineered with a gene that allows plants to tolerate glyphosate, nontolerant plants, including weeds, can't grow. Glyphosate has also been intentionally used on nontolerant crops, like oats, shortly before harvest, stopping photosynthesis and making the drying out process of the grain more efficient, though this use has declined in the last decade. Residues of the herbicide can also be detected on nontreated crops due to drift from treated crops.

In 2018, a slew of news outlets, including *CBS News, CNN, The Hill,* and others, raised the alarm over a report from the EWG finding trace amounts of the herbicide in several "children's" breakfast foods. Genetically engineered crops, known commonly as GMOs for *genetically modified organisms,* have been widely reviled, and glyphosate is one of the main GMO-related hot buttons. Opponents of the herbicide, many of whom call for a ban, say that it's responsible for a raft of health problems. Proponents say that glyphosate is one of the safest and most effective herbicides, that there is no compelling evidence that it's harmful to the general public, and that banning it would mean reverting to more caustic formulations.

When thinking of exposures to chemicals, there's an important distinction between acute and chronic toxicity. Our children's lives are basically an ongoing dynamic interaction involving the seas of molecules within them and surrounding them. This includes the molecules that are crucial in the body's processes, like metabolism, protein synthesis, and cognition. Toxicity is essentially the degree to which an exposure can disturb these bodily dynamics in some significant way that damages or harms an individual.

Acute toxicity looks at classical poisoning effects. LD50, where *LD* stands for *lethal dose*, is the amount of a substance taken all at once that results in the death of 50% of a group of test animals, and it's one way to measure the short-term poisoning potential of a chemical. The higher the LD50, which can be calculated for various routes of exposure, with skin and oral exposure among the most commonly measured, the lower the acute toxicity of a substance. Acute toxicity is largely outdated because the amount of a substance it would take to kill someone in one go is not particularly helpful as long as people keep harmful household chemicals out of the reach of young children. Scholars also note that classic LD50 experiments and the use of acute toxicity itself as a measure are problematic because fatality rates in subjects may vary in different experiments, different species and different individuals of the same species can react differently to the same substance, and it's unethical to kill a large number of lab animals, or any lab animals at all, depending on who you ask.

All the same, we know rough LD50 values for lots of substances. Water has an LD50 of 90,000 mg/kg: a hypothetical group of adult humans would have to consume roughly five or six liters of water all at once for half of them to die.

Let's compare the acute toxicity of glyphosate to caffeine, which many of us consider a gift from nature, and that kids consume in chocolate milk, soda, tea, or coffee. Because Layla Katiraee is a nerd of epic proportions, in 2019 she decided to figure out how much caffeine is safe for children per day. (Short answer: depending on their age and body weight, they can have some chocolate milk, a cup or two of tea, or other foods or drinks with a similar caffeine content relatively safely, though it's important to ensure that kids get enough sleep.)

Based on LD50, caffeine and vanillin (the compound that gives vanilla its flavor) are more acutely toxic than glyphosate. You would hypothetically need less pure caffeine or vanillin to poison someone than glyphosate—nearly thirty times less caffeine and over three times less vanillin. Rotenone, a naturally derived insecticide that was widely used in organic farming not long ago, has a lower estimated lethal dose than not only glyphosate, caffeine, and vanillin but also the insecticide Dichlorodiphenyltrichloroethane (DDT). And even more acutely toxic than DDT and rotenone is hydrogen cyanide, which is produced when the pits of peaches, apricots, and plums are chewed or crushed (so as natural as they are, don't put fruit pits in a smoothie).

Chronic toxicity measures are more useful than acute toxicity because they tell us the level of a substance that can cause harm with repeated exposures over time. These adverse effects include increased risk of disease, behavioral changes, reproductive effects, and others. The US Environmental Protection Agency (EPA) determines reference doses, or an estimate of the highest daily oral exposure of any substance, for humans, including "sensitive subgroups," that is "likely to be without an appreciable risk of deleterious effects during a lifetime." Though chronic toxicity estimates are known for many substances, reference doses have been most commonly determined for pesticides. These limits are calculated using formulas that include uncertainty factors, or anything that would warrant erring on the side of caution, like evidence that a certain chemical might affect some people more than others.

In addition to one-time poisoning effects, according to the available evidence on chronic toxicity, caffeine and vanillin are more toxic in the long term than glyphosate, meaning that, hypothetically, someone could ingest a higher dose of glyphosate daily than caffeine or vanillin without seeing adverse effects in a lifetime. (Incidentally, caffeine is also sometimes used as an insecticide. Though some insects, including some pollinators, can tolerate caffeine, and even get a buzz from it, it can kill or paralyze others.) I'd far rather have a dash of vanilla in my kids' cereal than glyphosate. At the same time, a trace amount of glyphosate in oats is not on my list of big concerns for my own children's well-being. To put things into perspective, the EPA threshold for glyphosate, which was set in 1993, is 2 mg/kg of body weight per day. According to its report (which wasn't peer-reviewed but simply published online), none of EWG's tested samples even came close to approaching those levels.

As it often goes, the Scary Substance in Children's Food or Other Products headlines were quickly followed by refutations along the lines of Actually, You Don't Need to Worry about Scary Substance in Kids' Food articles.

These refutations to the EWG's reported findings took issue with the threshold the organization set. EWG doesn't share much about its methodology, including where samples were obtained and whether they were obtained randomly. According to the EWG, several samples exceeded their threshold, including Cheerios Toasted Whole Grain Oat Cereal, which had readings of up to 530 ppb; and Quaker Old Fashioned Oats, which had readings of up to 1300 ppb. In short, according to EWG, several samples failed their test, and parents should be really worried if we care about our kids' health.

"Basically, the EWG threshold has to be set at one ten-thousandth of what the EPA has deemed to be safe for the trace amounts of glyphosate to register," wrote Susan Matthews, the executive editor for *Slate*. "Let's talk about what that means in terms of how much cereal you actually eat. The EWG threshold of 0.01 mg per day translates to a maximum of 160 ppb, given an assumed serving size of 60 grams, which is about 2 cups of cereal or ¾ cup of oatmeal. The parts per billion detected per food sample tested by EWG ranged from 10 to 1,300. So yes, some of them cross the EWG threshold. None crosses California's threshold, and none crosses the EPA threshold. In order to cross California's very conservative threshold, you'd need to eat 7½ cups of the worst kind of oatmeal a day. In order to cross the EPA threshold, you'd need to eat 100 times that."

A child would have to ingest a horror movie's worth of cereal or hummus every day before even approaching a toxic amount of glyphosate. In effect, even a toddler who *loves* toasted oat cereal and eats it all day every day is not in harm's way.

As for the fruits and veggies on the EWG's Dirty Dozen List, or any fruits and vegetables sold in the US for that matter, chemical residues are present in such low amounts that it would be impossible for a child to eat enough food to approach the EPA's thresholds. Beyond that, the protective effects of eating plenty of fruits and veggies—including organic or conventional, fresh, frozen, or canned—far exceed the risk of pesticide residues on any of them. Most children and adults in the United States do not consume enough fruits and vegetables and miss out on their important nutrients.

Evidence-based safe food-handling includes using separate cutting boards for vegetables and meats, cutting off and discarding damaged parts of fruits and vegetables, and removing the outer leaves of leafy produce such as cabbage or cauliflower. Washing fruits and vegetables under running water before eating minimizes agricultural chemical residues and rinsing firm produce like melons before cutting prevents the entry of pathogens from the surface. Washing items before peeling them so that bacteria and dirt from the skin don't get transferred is also not a bad idea. The risk of foodborne illness is lower for boiled and cooked foods, but safe handling can reduce risk if your kids like raw veggies.

The thing is, some substances are known to be harmful when present in minuscule amounts, especially to children, like lead in drinking water. But glyphosate isn't one of them, and the evidence for that is overwhelming. All of this tells me one thing: glyphosate in my kids' cereal and hummus doesn't earn a spot on my very long worry list, at least when it comes to my children's health.

The EPA is among a handful of agencies with cancer-classification systems for carcinogens. Its guidelines for carcinogen risk assessment sort substances into one of five categories for both inhalation and oral exposure: Carcinogenic to Humans, Likely to Be Carcinogenic to Humans, Suggestive Evidence of Carcinogenic Potential, Inadequate Information to Assess Carcinogenic Potential, or Not Likely to Be Carcinogenic to Humans. The EPA considers how strongly carcinogenic the chemical is, also known as its potency, its potential to cause cancer in lab animals, its potential to cause cancer in humans, the potential for human exposure, and the extent to which people might be exposed. They consider short-term studies, long-term cancer studies, studies of mutagenicity (or a substance's ability to induce genetic mutations), and more. They also make note of whether there are plausible modes of action for causing cancer. The cancer classification may be reevaluated as evidence accumulates, but the EPA's stance is that it does not have the resources to reevaluate every chemical regularly, and there is no reason to do so unless there is some new information that could change the basic understanding of that chemical. As for glyphosate, based on available data that it's been reviewing since 1974, the EPA determined that it is unlikely to be a human carcinogen in that "there are no risks of concern to human health when glyphosate is used in accordance with its current label." These categorizations are based on risk, not just hazard.

So where did the idea that glyphosate is supposedly cancer-causing originate? In large part, it comes from the International Agency for Research on Cancer or IARC, a specialized agency of the WHO based in Lyon, France. What's often confusing about the IARC is that the agency categorizes substances based on hazard and not risk.

IARC slots various agents, including occupational, lifestyle, and environmental exposures, into four possible categories. Group 1 is for established carcinogens, including smoking, asbestos, alcohol consumption, and processed meat. The next two tiers, 2A ("probably carcinogenic") and 2B ("possibly carcinogenic"), are for substances with a less certain causal relationship with cancer. Group 3 is for substances that can't be classified due to lack of data. There was once a fifth category, Group 4 ("probably not carcinogenic"), but they only ever slotted one agent into it—caprolactam, a compound used in the manufacture of synthetic fibers—and eliminated the category altogether in 2019.

If an agency, let's say the International Agency for Research on Cuts, similarly categorized agents that can cause cuts, then razor blades, scissors, printer paper, machetes, box cutters, kitchen knives, glassware, chain saws, katanas, toothbrushes, and guillotines would all be in Group 1 for items that are known to be "cut-causing to humans." But the risk of cuts from exposure to any of these hazards varies wildly, even though we know that all of them could potentially cause cuts in various situations. Like most other modern humans, my family keeps knives and glassware in our kitchen and unsharpened toothbrushes in our bathrooms, and we strongly believe that guillotines don't belong in the home.

One confusing piece is that all of these carcinogenic classifications are, again, not easily translated to individuals. They are based on the strength of evidence that these agents could cause additional cases of cancer in a population in some specific situation, not the degree of risk for one person. The International

Agency for Research on Cancer's Group 1, with over a hundred agents, including asbestos, processed meat, alcoholic beverages, certain infectious diseases, and sunlight, are billed as *carcinogenic to humans*. What this means is that we can be fairly sure that these agents have the potential to add beads to some people's multiple types of cancer jars in some situations.

Hazards in IARC's Group 2A are described as "probably carcinogenic to humans," which means that there's some evidence that they could cause cancer, but we can't be sure. Again, the word *probably* vaguely implies individual risk, but the classification isn't about individuals at all. Group 2B, "possibly carcinogenic to humans," may be "the most confusing one of all," according to Pulitzer Prize–winning science journalist Ed Yong. "What does 'possibly' even mean?" The lack of context about the risks or odds is misleading. Ultimately, "2B becomes a giant dumping ground for all the risk factors that IARC has considered, and could neither confirm nor fully discount as carcinogens. Which is to say: most things… But try telling someone unfamiliar with this that, say, power lines are 'possibly carcinogenic' and see what they take away from that." The practice of lumping risk factors into categories without including a description of their respective risks "practically invites people to view them as like-for-like," writes Yong. "And that inevitably led to misleading headlines like this one in the *Guardian*: 'Processed meats rank alongside smoking as cancer causes—WHO.'" Without context, IARC's classification says nothing about how processed meat compares to other Group 1 carcinogens like sunlight or formaldehyde. My youngest kid loves salami, and while we don't feed it to him every single day, he eats around one Italian sub per week on average. By contrast, I certainly wouldn't give him permission to smoke a cigarette.

The EPA has reviewed both EWG's and IARC's statements on glyphosate and affirmed that the herbicide is safe when used as intended and not actually carcinogenic to children and adults who eat oatmeal and hummus. The EWG suggesting that the IARC's 2017 categorization of glyphosate in Group 2A—which includes drinking very hot beverages and night-shift work that disrupts the circadian rhythm—means that it causes cancer in kids eating cereal is far more than a stretch.

Among substances that I personally worry about more than glyphosate is radon, which the EPA categorizes as a known human carcinogen and that the IARC includes in its carcinogenic to humans Group 1 category. Radon is thought to account for up to 50% of the public's exposure to naturally occurring sources of radiation in many countries. Experts believe that radon causes up to 14% of lung cancers in countries around the world and causes most of the lung cancers that aren't a result of cigarette smoking. This naturally occurring radioactive gas mostly comes from bedrock and has a tendency to accumulate indoors. Testing of radon levels and its decay products in the air is the only way to know the level of exposure to radon, high levels of which can have a major impact on air quality in homes, schools, workplaces, and other indoor spaces. Levels can vary significantly within the same neighborhood, so a low level measured in the building next door doesn't mean that someone's home is in the clear. The EPA's website says that radon "is a health hazard with a simple solution" and provides resources to obtain discounted radon test kits. It also provides details on hiring credentialed mitigation service providers, who vent radon from below the dwelling into the outside air so that the gas doesn't accumulate inside. We found that the radon level in our home was elevated. Getting it mitigated isn't cheap—we paid just under a thousand dollars in 2023. So while the solution may be relatively simple, it is not equitable.

The fear-driven movements in the food and health spheres, like the clean-living trend, are rooted in some very justified concerns. There are plenty of facts to show that we *should* worry about our kids' breakfasts. Children are bombarded with predatory marketing of added sugars, and far too many kids are food insecure. Misconceptions and lack of scientific thinking about chemicals and chemistry aren't the fundamental drivers of free-from claims. Rather, making informed choices based on our values is overwhelming, confusing, and highly inaccessible, especially when added to the existing challenges of parenthood in the twenty-first century. So turning to labels to assuage the anxiety is understandable. Research suggests that no-no lists and free-from claims reflect a lack of trust in the food system, other industries, and the government, a craving for transparency and authenticity, and a desire to be empowered and heard. These underlying desires make sense, but taking actions that make us feel like we've made the responsible choice don't necessarily help us. My fellow SciParents and I have realized that avoiding proxies that symbolize harm—like the ingredients on no-no lists—as stand-ins for what we're really worried about doesn't protect our children or help them thrive. Yes, the food, pharmaceutical, and many other industries continue to cause harm, and too often, the government fails to mitigate it. But avoiding the Dirty Dozen isn't the answer. There's nothing about foods sold as organic that make them safer or healthier for kids who eat them. For all of the energy and time we expend to scour Dirty Dozen and no-no lists, what do we gain?

In some places, communities are fighting to take control of their food access. In my city of Madison in 2019, entrepreneur Mariam Maldonado opened Luna's Groceries with the help of a grant from the city to improve retail food access in the Allied Drive–Dunn's Marsh neighborhood. There were no grocery stores there for years, and pedestrians couldn't walk to small stores outside the community safely with the huge intersection nearby. Now, residents with no vehicle, and no convenient bus route to an area with a grocery store, can purchase fresh food with "an inventory that is built to the input of that neighborhood," Maldonado told *Wisconsin Watch* in 2022.

For some families, community farming initiatives have been one way to tangibly empower communities, like the Urban Growers Collective in Chicago. With eight urban farms on eleven acres of land, predominantly located on Chicago's South Side, the collective aims to address the inequities and structural racism that exist in the food system on a local level. The collective works to provide jobs and mitigate food insecurity and limited access to "affordable, culturally affirming, and nutritionally dense food." As part of the Chicago Food Policy Action Council, they also help facilitate the development of policies to improve access to affordable food grown through environmentally sustainable practices for the city's residents.

Even with local initiatives like these, we still have to push systems to change on a large scale for all children to thrive. **The food system is among those that shift the onus to individuals to take control of their kids' health, while glossing over the fact that institutions bear the bulk of the responsibility to improve outcomes.** Our stress levels are understandably high in a world where systems are failing our children so spectacularly. The chemicals in our lives are a fulcrum around which this stress revolves, driving the desire for a clean life. Those with ample privilege and buying power assuage their anxieties by making comforting, seemingly important choices in the marketplace. That's why, for all categories of consumer goods, there are alternatives that marketers position as more natural, safe, or clean. It can feel soothing to avoid any scary thing that seems avoidable, whether or not this action reduces risk.

Choosing to avoid certain chemicals or other substances can be benign, beneficial, or even crucial. For instance, fragrance-free detergents or personal-care products can help people with sensitivities to fragrance. Certain people born with the genetic disease phenylketonuria (PKU), those with advanced liver disease, and pregnant individuals with very high levels of the amino acid phenylalanine in the blood should avoid the artificial sweetener aspartame, which contains phenylalanine. (These folks also need to minimize eggs, dairy, milk, beans, and nuts, because they all contain phenylalanine, and consume a special supplemental formula that contains protein without this specific amino acid.) And among the most prominent examples is people with celiac disease avoiding gluten, a protein that naturally occurs in certain grains like wheat.

But choosing what seems like a safer alternative for what seems like a bad chemical can sometimes have very real negative consequences. For instance, unregulated homemade infant formula, which some people use because they fear the chemicals in store-bought formula, can seriously harm a baby. Treating bacterial infections with natural remedies instead of prescribed antibiotics, which some people do because of selective aversion to mainstream medical advice, can lead to some nasty complications, like strep throat progressing to a life-threatening condition or ear infections progressing to permanent hearing loss. Avoiding vaccines because of the fear of chemicals brushes over the increased risk of catching and spreading a vaccine-preventable illness.

Using homeopathic remedies sold in drugstores is a waste of money at best—homeopathy is not medicine but a system of pseudoscience that hinges on the idea that a substance that causes symptoms of a disease can cure similar symptoms, or the *like cures like* doctrine. Homeopathic remedies are made using homeopathic dilution during which the selected substance is repeatedly diluted until the final product contains no detectable amount of the supposed active ingredient. Often not even a single molecule of the original substance can be expected to remain in the product. Between each dilution, homeopaths may hit or shake the product, claiming this makes the concoction "remember" the original substance after its removal. All available relevant scientific knowledge contradicts homeopathy. None of the homeopathic products marketed in drugstores have an effect on any known disease. There are no FDA-approved products that are labeled as homeopathic.

Yet, there are widely available homeopathic remedies sold in major US drugstores for everything from flu-like symptoms to muscle soreness to help falling asleep. And these products are displayed alongside actual medicine proven to have modes of action in the body. They can seem like a sensible way to help your child or yourself feel better, but these products don't do anything.

The claims that the sellers of these products make, along with the idea that homeopathy is more natural or gentle than Big Pharma offerings, can be compelling.

There is perhaps "nothing worse than your child being in pain, even when you know it's temporary," fellow SciParent Anastasia Bodnar pointed out in a post about teething remedies. A few months into infancy, intense and prolonged crying is often chalked up to cutting baby teeth. "It's no surprise that parents through the ages have reached for any remedies that might relieve their child's teething," she wrote. Dealing with the excessive drooling and bawling that's often associated with teething is an age-old rite of early parenthood. "People have tried remedies from slicing the gums to rubbing rabbit brains on them, and obviously, have failed," Bodnar writes. What many parents don't know is that what we perceive as symptoms of teething in our babies can seem "much worse than they are" and may not actually be due to teething itself. While it may be uncomfortable, evidence suggests that the eruption of baby teeth themselves isn't as painful as we tend to assume. Since teething happens during a time of rapid change in a baby's life, crying, fever, vomiting, diarrhea, or sleep disturbances are often attributed to teething. This is a big reason that parents "still reach for remedies" for teething "that range from unhelpful to harmful," including applying small amounts of hard liquor to the gums or the use of homeopathic teething tablets. Fever, vomiting, or diarrhea could be a sign of infection, and a parent should contact their healthcare provider if an infant has these symptoms. For any potential discomfort for teething, the FDA recommends two options: gently rub or massage the child's gums, or give them a teething ring made of firm rubber. The teething ring shouldn't be frozen solid, and, as always, supervise the chewing to prevent choking.

What researchers call the placebo by proxy effect, in which a caretaker feels like their child's (or even a pet's) symptoms have improved simply because there's been an intervention, is often at play with babies and nonverbal children. But what we think of as symptoms of teething, or of colic in earlier infancy, are often subjective. As an added stressor, babies' bouts of crying aren't easy to attribute to anything specific, especially if they're still crying after being fed, rocked, changed, and held. And whose heart can tolerate their upset little wailing faces? Parents' perceptions of these symptoms are sensitive to numerous placebo effects. Babies can cry a lot for any or no reason, and when they stop, it's tempting to attribute it to something specific, especially if you did something specific in the hopes of soothing your little one. This is not to say that the placebo effect is necessarily a bad thing. I once regularly spritzed a little homemade Scary Spray to keep the nightmares away when my kids were young enough to buy it. It seemed to help them settle down at night as part of their bedtime routine when they were little. The question is always whether the risk of exposing a child to something is worth the benefit. The negligible risk of spraying a bit of saline solution in the air to help my little one sleep—and the eventual learning experience when they realized that there is no proven fear-repelling spray—seemed worth it to me.

Ultimately, worrying about relatively benign chemicals can distract us from other toxic exposures that are particularly risky for our children. What's tricky about EWG specifically is that its spurious campaigns like the Dirty Dozen and the glyphosate in cereal report overshadow the group's work on some chemicals that should concern us.

Consider lead. Soil naturally contains low levels of lead, but mining, smelting, and refining have resulted in substantial increases in lead levels elsewhere in the environment where humans are more readily exposed. When lead is released into the air from industrial sources or small-aircraft ignition, it can travel long distances before settling on the ground. EWG has warned against lead in drinking water, and it's absolutely right on this. The EPA and experts worldwide agree. A naturally occurring element found in small amounts in the Earth's crust, in fossil fuels, and previously found in certain types of gasoline, paints, pipes, and other products, lead is hazardous to our health. Evidence presented in a 2022 research article published in the *Proceedings of the National Academy of Sciences* found that millions of adults were exposed to high levels of lead as children. While these exposures were deemed harmless at the time, data accrued since then reveal that these exposures likely disrupted healthy development on a population level, resulting in subtle effects on important outcomes, like cognition, fine motor skills, and emotional regulation, that "may influence the trajectory of a person's life (e.g., their educational attainment, health, wealth, and happiness)."

Unlike glyphosate, it's important to measure the presence of lead in parts per billion. In 1991, the EPA set a rule replacing the previous limit of 50 ppb in water for lead, measured at the entry point to the distribution system, with the current limit of 15 ppb. Lead exposure can happen through contaminated food or water or from dishes or glasses that contain lead. People can also inhale lead dust from lead-based paint. Exposure to lead during pregnancy can be particularly harmful, as can childhood exposure. Kids' growing bodies absorb more lead than adults, and their brains and nervous systems are more sensitive to the damaging effects. Babies have additional exposure from putting their hands and other objects contaminated with lead from dust or soil into their mouths. Even extremely low levels of lead in a child's blood can result in harm to organ systems, behavior and learning problems, slow growth, anemia, and seizures.

If more than 10% of tap samples exceed the lead action level of 15 parts per billion, then water systems are required to take additional action. The EPA has a "maximum contaminant" goal of zero for lead in drinking water, but these goals are not enforceable. Like other harmful exposures that disproportionately affect marginalized children, there are vast disparities in lead exposure and clear socioeconomic disparities in blood lead levels, with Black and low-income children the most affected in the United States. The city of Flint, Michigan—which in April of 2014 changed its water supply source from Lake Huron to the Flint River, causing water distribution pipes to leach lead and other contaminants into municipal drinking water—was among US cities that helped get these water crises on the map. But the fight for safe water for all children is far from over. It wasn't until late in 2022 that the EPA released its first-ever agency-wide "Strategy to Reduce Lead Exposures and Disparities in US Communities." This strategy, which includes updating lead service lines, cleaning up construction projects where lead contamination is known to be high, and connecting communities with resources that can reduce lead exposure, is promising, but there's a long road ahead.

As we've seen time and again, factors that harm children's health converge to compound the negative impacts on the well-being of the most marginalized. Scientists know that food security and nutrition are major protectors against harm from lead. Children with full stomachs absorb less lead than those whose stomachs are empty. Diets with plenty of nutrients, especially calcium, iron, and vitamin C, help minimize the effects of lead exposure. Rather than worrying about the Dirty Dozen, imagine what we could do if we put our energy into fighting for food security for all.

In the home, in addition to a nutritious diet, the best ways to prevent harm from lead include getting a residence tested for lead if it was built before 1978; regular washing of hands, bottles, pacifiers, and toys; letting tap water run for one minute before using it; using only cold water for drinking, cooking, and mixing baby formula (lead from pipes is more prone to leaching into water when hot); regularly cleaning surfaces that collect dust with wet methods (not dry dusters); and not using imported pottery to store or serve food. Although someone's home may be free of lead-based paint, your child could be exposed elsewhere, especially if they spend time in a building built before 1978. Check whether your school inspects its facilities for lead hazards. If you suspect that your child has been exposed to lead, it's worth having them tested, even if they aren't showing any symptoms.

EWG has also warned against PFAS, which stands for *per-and polyfluoroalkyl substances*—a group of manufactured chemicals that have been used in industry and consumer products since the 1940s because they are durable and resistant to stains, heat, grease, and water. The EPA, the CDC, the AAP, and the WHO are among those who agree that PFAS are a public-health concern, especially for children. PFAS are concerning to me, albeit in a different way than lead is. These chemicals fall under the broader category of Persistent Organic Pollutants (POPs), which are pesticides or insecticides, solvents, pharmaceuticals, and industrial chemicals that include DDT, polychlorinated biphenyls (PCBs), and dioxins. Although some POPs arise naturally, like from volcanic activity or forest fires, most are synthetic. One major issue with POPs including PFAS is that many break down very slowly and can accumulate in humans, animals, plants, other organisms, and the environment over time, which is why they're referred to as "forever chemicals."

There are thousands of different PFAS, some of which have been more widely used and studied than others. For instance, perfluorooctanoic acid (PFOA) and perfluorooctane sulfonate (PFOS), with several industrial uses including clothing treatments, firefighting foams, and carpets, are two of the most widely used and studied types of PFAS chemicals. PFOA and PFOS have been replaced in the United States with other PFAS in recent years. And unfortunately, PFAS are as close to everywhere on Earth as a substance can be, so much so that Bernstein says that she "would be more surprised if something wasn't contaminated with PFAS." Scientists know that PFAS are harmful in some way and have been contributing to health problems for decades, but they still don't know exactly how. There's evidence to suggest that exposure to certain PFAS at high levels may have reproductive effects like decreased fertility or complications during pregnancy like preeclampsia, low birth weight, developmental effects in children, accelerated puberty, bone variations, or behavior issues. They may also contribute to increased risk of some cancers, reduced immune response, including reduced vaccine response, interference with the activity of hormones, increased cholesterol levels, and other conditions. Whether and how PFAS exposure affects the risk of various infections, including COVID-19, is still an open question. It's challenging for scientists to pin down the health effects in more detail because there are so many kinds of PFAS with varying effects and toxicity levels, and most studies focus on a limited number of them.

In part, the problem is that the government hasn't been able to tackle all of the thousands of PFAS in a unified way—or hasn't prioritized doing so. More and more experts are calling for governments and industries to treat these chemicals as one class. When venting about this with the SciParents, Anastasia Bodnar points out that there are "a lot of things that we do badly because we do it case-by-case instead of holistically" when it comes to groups of chemicals like PFAS that have similar structures and properties.

It's not just PFAS. With all kinds of chemicals, evidence that one might be bad too often leads to what toxicologists call *regrettable substitutions* with something similar—think of the series of studies that famously led to the removal of Bisphenol A (BPA), a chemical used to harden plastics since the 1950s, from several industrially produced plastics, including children's sippy cups and bottles in 2012. Several manufacturers replaced BPA with analogs, and research has since suggested that these substitutions, often used in products that boast BPA-free labels, probably aren't any safer.

In 2023, the EPA under the Biden–Harris administration announced its first-ever national standard to address PFAS exposures in communities, including a drinking-water standard for six types of PFAS. It's a start, but let's not forget that there are thousands of PFAS. Though there has been increased attention to these chemicals in the last few years, scientists have known for the better part of the last century that they are not good for our children or for the planet, yet "we only regulate one at a time, doing the same thing over and over and expecting the outcome to be different," Bernstein vents. Though there has been a concerted push for stricter regulations, companies are still producing PFAS.

What concerns me most about PFAS is the disparities in how people are exposed and affected, that companies still use them, and that cleaning up this contamination in any significant way will require steep global investment in technological solutions, and even then, it is likely to take decades to make a dent. In any case, we better get it done. These chemicals are going to remain everywhere for hundreds to thousands of years unless there's a definitive and coordinated effort, and I know that we as progressive parents don't want future generations left with this mess. Again, those who bear most of the amorphous harm from PFAS are the most marginalized.

Francesca Hong points out that our hometown is among many in America and in the world where we find higher levels of pollutants in areas with mobile homes and rentals. In Madison, this includes residential areas closer to the Dane County airport. The distribution of Black and brown people, and those with low incomes, is "directly correlated" with toxic exposures, she explains.

There's not a whole lot we can do as individuals to protect our kids from PFAS right now, but, as with lead, there are a few meaningful actions we can take while pushing for systemic change. First, find out if PFAS are in your drinking water. In the US, some local water utilities will have something to say about how they may be addressing PFAS and information about the results of testing for these chemicals in your municipality's drinking water, but not all of them have this information. For those who want to check the PFAS levels in their private well water, the EPA recommends contacting your state for a listing of certified laboratories using EPA-developed testing methods. Certain types of treatment technologies or in-home water filters that are certified to lower the levels of some PFAS are an option. Studies show limited absorption of PFAS through the skin, so showering or bathing are not considered significant sources of exposure.

Some of the actions we can take are often easier said than done; for instance, avoid occupational exposures like touching concentrated products in chemical-manufacturing facilities or breathing PFAS in the air at work as much as possible. Avoid living near current or former military bases or industrial facilities that use PFAS. If you live in an area with PFAS concerns, use ready-to-feed baby formula or mix formula using alternative water sources that do not have PFAS, and drink and cook with safe water if you're lactating. Check local fish-consumption guidelines before eating locally sourced fish or seafood or wild game. Since PFAS and other chemicals like lead can build up in dust, regular mopping, wet-dusting, and vacuuming of surfaces can reduce exposure. Reduce or avoid nonstick cookware, and consider safer alternatives like stainless steel and cast iron. Consider avoiding stain-resistant carpets and upholstery. Reduce exposure to fast food and take-out containers, even those that claim to be eco-friendly, since it's hard to tell which ones have coatings with PFAS. Not going to lie, we get takeout fairly regularly.

The SciParents also worry about flame retardants (many of which fall under the category of POPs). They are common in many types of consumer and industrial products and have been in global use since the 1970s, but there's evidence to suggest that industry lobbyists have exaggerated the need for these chemicals. These are added to manufactured goods like children's clothing, electronics, and furniture to prevent or slow the spread of fire, but their fire-safety benefit is unclear, and there are several potential health effects that are concerning. When there is a fire, flame retardants produce toxic gases, which has also led to opposition from the International Association of Fire Fighters because of concern over the high rates of cancers in the fire service.

Much of the data that tell us about the health effects of fire retardants come from what the Michigan Department of Agriculture has called "the most costly and disastrous accidental contamination ever to occur in United States agriculture." In the early 1970s, the Michigan Chemical Corporation accidentally shipped several hundred pounds of flame retardant polybrominated biphenyls (PBBs) in place of a nutritional supplement to a livestock feed mill. As a result, nearly 10 million residents of the state's lower peninsula consumed contaminated meat, milk, and eggs before the company realized its toxic mistake. Since the voluntary phaseout of PBBs started in 2004, other flame retardants have replaced them, but these replacements aren't necessarily safer. In yet another case of regrettable substitutions, these chemicals have similar profiles for persistence, bioaccumulation, and toxicity.

Researchers think that this PBB disaster could have contributed to the development of cancer in some of those with high exposure, a higher likelihood of abnormal thyroid levels in exposed workers, higher rates of miscarriage during pregnancy in the adult pregnant children of those with high exposure, and higher rates of genital or urinary conditions. Human health effects at lower levels of exposure are unclear, but animal studies suggest that they may have effects on the thyroid, neurodevelopment, liver, and reproductive system.

Since the benefits of flame retardants are dubious, Bernstein is among toxicologists who say that we should have "a lower risk tolerance for the use of these chemicals" and "should question whether they are necessary for each application." If possible, she suggests avoiding flame retardants in children's clothing: new clothes with flame retardants often have tags that say so. A Google search can help identify brands of furniture and other products that do not use any flame retardants, not just those that have replaced one with another.

The risk from POPs is relatively low for those with the privilege of maximizing their families' protective exposures. **"I'm not particularly worried about my family's risk" from pesticides, flame retardants, processed meat, grilling, or other things that can add a bead to a risk jar, Bernstein explains. She often encourages parents to think of any exposure within "the entire landscape" of our exposures.** The risk landscape is full of modifiable and nonmodifiable risk factors that impact our health in big and small ways. Those with the means to do so can control some of the bigger risk factors in their families' lives, knowing that it'll help reduce their likelihood of a slew of health problems. **We can protect against the effects of many of the harmful exposures with smaller impacts that we can't change by focusing on the evidence-based modifiable protective exposures with big impacts, like eating lots of fruits and vegetables, having fulfilling relationships, not smoking, prioritizing mental health, being physically active, and so on.**

As a rule, even in situations where the SciParents are not worried about our own families' exposure to potentially harmful chemicals, we still worry about the people who work directly with them, communities with high levels of exposure, and persistence in the environment. Unfortunately, there are so many potentially harmful chemicals and other exposures that are stealthy and don't appear on lists of substances that supposedly clean brands proudly don't use. Consider stress. When it comes to the chemicals we worry about, the chemical pathways that stress triggers in parents and in children definitely make the cut. We live in a brutal world, and we know that childhood stress and trauma harm health and well-being throughout life. From the alarming and disparate increase of heat exposure, which global warming has exacerbated to noise pollution to air quality, so many of the worst hazards are out of the control of individual parents and families. Industries wield no-no lists to convince parents that their kid's health is in their hands, robbing us of our agency and energy. When we're distracted by the MSGs and the glyphosates of the chemical world, we have little bandwidth to fight against the most harmful chemicals and systemic forces that overwhelmingly shape our well-being. Worrying about living a clean life can distract us from holding systems accountable for the well-being of children who experience toxic exposures, not from strawberries, oatmeal, or hummus but from the very places where they live, learn, and sleep. Putting the burden on individuals' choices allows institutions to make surface-level changes without addressing the root of disparities—injustice.

7

greenwashing our children's future

Driving around the United States makes one thing clear. Not only do we not have flying cars but the electric-vehicle revolution hasn't happened. Despite highway expansion, traffic persists. Cars spew harmful pollutants. Children and families living in poverty, near busy intersections, or without a dependable ride in rural areas or in unwalkable cities deal with a higher risk of pedestrian accidents and fatalities, added exposure to pollutants, and a lack of access to groceries, health care, and other needs. Optimistic projections suggest that the US could see nearly a trillion dollars in public-health benefits by 2050 if several more states invest in widespread electric-car-charging infrastructure and eliminate the sales of gasoline- and diesel-powered vehicles by 2035. That rosy dream—in which everyone has their own truly sustainable form of personal transportation, the air is clear, and the future is bright—overlooks the most marginalized children today, who continue to bear the worst exposures to pollution and the effects of living near highways, or living without reliable transportation while we wait for the electric-vehicle revolution.

We know that climate change due to greenhouse gas (GHG) emissions from human activity is a surging global catastrophe. In 2021, carbon dioxide (CO_2) accounted for 79% of all US greenhouse gas emissions from human activities, including the burning of fossil fuels and other biological materials. As a natural part of the Earth's carbon cycle, the element constantly suffuses the atmosphere, oceans, soil, and living things. Humans have upended the equilibrium between carbon *sources*, which release more carbon than they capture, and *sinks*, like forests and soil, which capture more than they release, thrusting us into planetary chaos. The Earth's intrinsic greenhouse effect is a result of naturally occurring GHGs in the atmosphere that trap heat from the sun; this is a big part of what makes our planet habitable. Naturally occurring water vapor is technically the most abundant greenhouse gas and is responsible for about half of the planet's greenhouse effect. The evidence suggests that water vapor produced directly by human activity contributes only negligibly to the water vapor in the atmosphere. Indirectly, the effects of global warming from human emissions of other GHGs—including carbon dioxide, methane (CH_4), nitrous oxide (N_2O), and fluorinated gases—add to the base level of water vapor in the atmosphere, exacerbating the effects of human emissions.

Earth Day, founded by the US senator and later two-term governor of Wisconsin, Gaylord Nelson, has been held annually on April 22 since 1970 when millions participated in the event around the United States. It went global in 1990, with an estimated 200 million people participating in over 140 nations. The story goes that Senator Nelson was inspired to create Earth Day upon the sight from an airplane of a devastating 800-square-mile oil slick in the Santa Barbara Channel following the oil spill in 1969. On April 22, 2017, rallies for the inaugural March for Science were held worldwide to coincide with Earth

Day. I was one of the speakers at the Madison rally that year, which also included Bassam Shakhashiri, a chemistry professor at UW-Madison, noted science educator, and advocate for science education, and Tia Nelson, an environmental activist and the daughter of Gaylord Nelson. As spectacular and moving as Earth Day has been as a global movement with its roots in my home state, I can't help but think sadly of my childhood friends. Back then, we believed that celebrating Earth Day could save us and that the trees we planted and the trash we collected would ensure our bright futures. On April 22, 2023, my own Earth Day baby turned ten years old. I smiled, brimming with love as he blew out his candles, feeling thankful for our safe home and for three generations of our family celebrating under one roof, not knowing what the future holds, and with a pang of guilt for our relatively soft existence at that moment.

As profound as they've been, all of the Earth Days over the span of half a century have not prevented the global catastrophe that rages around us. Scientists warn that the world will almost certainly reach record temperatures by 2027. There have been dire effects on health, food security, water levels, and biodiversity with more to come. We lurch together into increasingly uncharted territory. World leaders have warned of the urgent need to limit the global average temperature to well below 2°C above preindustrial levels, with a target limit of 1.5°C (or 2.7°F) to avoid the most cataclysmic consequences. To prevent breaching the limit, GHG emissions will need to peak by 2025 at the latest and decline 43% by 2030. In other words, we may be able to avoid it, but just barely, and with far too many casualties, even with a most gargantuan effort. To undertake the accelerated action required to limit warming, nations agreed to cut greenhouse gas emissions as part of the Paris Agreement, which entered into force in November of 2016. Things since then have been dicey.

I can't help but think that we are channeling that iconic smiling cartoon dog wearing a brimmed hat, calmly sitting

at a table with a cup of coffee, assuring himself that "This is fine" as the room goes up in flames. The dog went viral in 2014, with its pleasant-yet-terrified grin in K. C. Green's famous 2013 webcomic "On Fire." It quickly came to symbolize any situation in which things have gotten so dire that our brains refuse to comprehend reality. The first few panels of the comic are often taken out of context; the scene usually appears without the last four panels of the strip. In the second half, the dog takes a sip of coffee and continues via speech bubble, "I'm okay with the events that are unfolding currently." He pauses, takes another sip, smiles, and continues, "Things are going to be okay." In the final panel, the flames engulf the still-eerily grinning character as he suffocates and burns alive, eyes bulging. Ostensibly, things are not at all "okay" nor is the poor dog "fine."

For its part, the US EPA, with its momentum blunted under the Trump administration, has also been channeling the dog. It wasn't until well after the emergency was out of hand that the agency issued a flurry of new proposed standards for pollution in the water and air, vehicle emissions, and more.

Three years after the webcomic went viral, K. C. Green created a new version, in which the dog snaps out of his smiling stupor just in time to scream, "This is not fine!! Oh my God everything's on fire!" As he runs around the room putting out the flames with a fire extinguisher, he shouts, "There was no reason to let it last this long and get this bad." In the final two panels, he sits, still very much alive, but worn out and in despair, in a scorched room.

Some parents can't ignore the fire because they haven't had a choice. For Shaina Oliver and her children, who live just south of the Suncor refinery in northeast Denver, Colorado, the air is constantly toxic, making it hard to breathe. A tribal member of the Navajo Nation from Shiprock, New Mexico, Oliver grew more aware of the impact of environmental disasters on her tribe in 2015 after toxic mine wastewater spilled into the Animas and San Juan Rivers. Struck with a sense of responsibility to do her part "as a mother, aunt, sister, descendant, and survivor of genocide," she became an advocate for the environment and Indigenous peoples' rights. With the help of the Moms Clean Air Force, a nonprofit environmental-advocacy group that works to protect children from air pollution and climate change, she began to testify at EPA hearings and in support of environmental bills at the US Capitol.

People in Oliver's community are "living through it and they're living next to it," she tells me on a call in 2022. Nobody, including children, can escape the terrible effects of pollution. "It's just such an energy drain to breathe in air toxics, and it has a tremendous impact on your body." When canvasing, she's met people who use oxygen tanks, who have heart disease, high blood pressure, asthma, diabetes, or cancer. Oliver tells me that her friend and fellow organizer has been taking her mom and aunt to chemotherapy appointments while dealing with a recent death in the family of leukemia, and even her dog dying of cancer. Oliver met a man who lost his wife and his son to cancer and continues to live in the area. Most are Spanish-speaking families, she explains, while some are Black community members "that have been pushed to live" here because "this is where the last of the affordable housing exists in Colorado right now," and even that is "still pretty high for affordable housing prices." This "environmental segregation of our housing" affects Black and brown people, immigrants, and low-income families who are "forced" to live next to these highways. "We continue to be that sacrifice" for "not just white communities but privileged communities that are at a higher income status" and who "don't have to live next to highways, don't have to live next to Suncor refineries," she explains. "But this is where our families are pushed." Families "end up next to Suncor because they couldn't find anywhere else to live." Some "are willing to camp out" and to "be homeless rather than live next to Suncor refinery," and "that is environmental injustice."

In Navajo stories, the air has always been revered as sacred and life-giving. Erasing Indigenous knowledge is what got us into this situation, Oliver says. The root cause of the climate crisis is "a nation that operates under anti-Native Americanism," which goes hand in hand with "a health crisis." Oliver engages with her community through health. "My grandfather was one of those uranium miners in the '60s who mined uranium without protective gear," she tells me. "The Navajo Nation and those people that were working in those mines, they weren't told about the health risks of mining uranium." Now, more than half a century later, community members who move near Suncor aren't told that their housing cost is lower "because it could be harmful to your children's health," and that, growing up in what she calls a "sacrifice zone," these kids "could die" before their parents. Oliver's community doesn't "have a lot more advocates for health," she says because "people have not had time to advocate in public spaces. People are working." There's often a message that "we need more" folks in the community to speak out, but you can't expect people to "be where they can't be." These people are service laborers experiencing "a segregation of work careers." They "don't choose to be in the service industry." Ultimately, class inequity "leaves us out of the decision-making" because there's "no time to be a part of that process. It gives us no time to really correlate what's going on in our community" with "how it's impacting my family," she says. She works to "bring their voices to the table" because they can't be there themselves. "I mean, we shouldn't have to tell our public leaders how to protect public health and environmental safety," Oliver vents. These leaders "took on that position of leadership to protect both public health and the environment." Oliver chuckles in frustration. "Why can't they provide a public health environment in the first place?" Industry "is ignoring and sidestepping our right to our health." She doesn't mince words when asked about the widespread messaging that parents should simply "take control of" their kids' health. "We should have more control of our health, but we don't. And if we could, we would." Until then, she and her fellow activists fight industry to put an end to these "sacrifice zones" and their deadly effects on children and families.

It's no wonder that climate grief is real, as climate activist and author Mary Annaïse Heglar often points out. "People used to ask me: 'What gives you hope?'" she recounts in a 2021 essay in *The Nation*. "I, like many other climate folks, found that question obnoxious." The question assumes that climate advocates have hope, she explains, "and it demands that we perform it for the audience." But she can't tell people that everything will be okay because it's not okay for a lot of people, which often leads her to "wallow in despair." These emotions are uncomfortable, but at the same time, she takes comfort in the fact that she can still experience them. "I never want to be the person who can look at so much suffering in this world and feel fine. It hurts because it's supposed to," Heglar insists. It's part of our humanity.

How do we honor our humanity, snap out of the stupor, and put out the fire? I'm still working on figuring it out, and so are a lot of other parents I know, and there's no simple answer. A big contributor to the collective stupor is one of our greatest nemeses as progressive parents—that old and omnipresent systemic urge to put the onus on individual choices to ensure children's well-being and to save the world. Starting in grade school, we're told that when you realize that a fire is too big to put out yourself, it's time to call the fire department. But what happens when the fire fighters don't come? What if you hear sirens in the distance but they're always tied up elsewhere? It's bleak for a lot of parents, and sometimes saying "this is fine" helps us get through our days while also helping our kids get through theirs. Most parents don't have the energy, time, or money for a lot more than that. For those with the bandwidth, making green choices can feel like playing a part in saving the Earth. It's certainly a lot more pleasant than staring reality in the face while screaming hopelessly into the abyss. Viral stories of low- or even no-waste parenting—including one family that famously reduced their household trash to a single jar of odds and ends for a whole year—are remarkable. But even as we strive to consume and waste less, reducing our individual trash from an average of nearly five pounds per day for Americans to a single jar in a year isn't attainable for most and may not be worth the strife. While we should do our best to reduce waste, sometimes we have to dispose of things. There's no shame in that. As Jenny Splitter put it in 2022, "I sometimes look at zero-waste Instagram and wonder if twelve different ways to repurpose your empty dental floss package is really a thing we need to spend time on."

Some say that the greenest choice is to not have kids at all. Yes, it makes sense to worry about our youth growing up in a burning world, inheriting a scorched planet, and, as a result, suffering and dying young. The concept of the personal carbon footprint has become increasingly coupled with concerns about the global human population in ways that can seem benign and even logical: each person's carbon footprint contributes to global warming, so the math in favor of less reproduction adds up. But it is everyone's human right to consider becoming a parent, including the layer of complexity that climate change adds to that consideration, and to do so if they so choose. Deciding not to have kids for any reason is totally valid. At the same time, while it can seem like a matter of simple math on its surface, the emphasis in some circles on population growth and its relationship to climate change enters eugenics territory and is not worth legitimizing.

Regarding the environment and sustainability, the ultimate dream of progressive parents is two-pronged. The first is to protect all children right now from the consequences of environmental destruction and global warming, and the

second is to stop the assault on our planet and begin to heal it. Those in the trenches fighting for all kids to thrive, even in a scorched world, are tenacious, but the burden is heavy. What can progressive parents do—including those who can't be in the trenches per se but who want to help as best as they can—to take on even a small amount of this burden?

First, we need to center equity and justice in informing actions. Climate change disproportionately impacts poor and marginalized people worldwide, and low-income countries deal with the worst impacts even though they have contributed very little to the causes. In the same vein, though it was founded with noble objectives, environmental activism was also founded on inequity. "The white environmentalist climate space" is a "self-absolving field" because it ignores "the impacts of colonization" on climate change, says Victor Lopez-Carmen, the aspiring pediatrician and advocate for Indigenous children's rights. Those who dominate environmentalism have "created an entire field dedicated to maintaining their privilege" even as our planet burns rather than taking responsibility and doing what needs to be done.

We know that some nations in the global North have been predominantly responsible for climate change. As a result, in places like Pakistan, India, Afghanistan, and Bangladesh, hundreds of millions of children face what UNICEF calls an "extremely high risk" of the impacts of the climate crisis, which compound the effects of poverty and chronic malnourishment. Add to this the impact of energy poverty: hundreds of millions worldwide live without electricity, and over 2 billion still use inefficient or harmful cooking systems. Devastating floods wash away schools, homes, and health-care facilities. Widespread damage to water systems leaves families with contaminated water. The question of how much the wealthiest nations and other entities owe the most vulnerable looms large. That has led to a push for what some call climate reparations, which would include payments for loss and damage. The idea is that countries, private corporations, and other entities whose GHG emissions have been highest over the years would be held accountable, take steps to elucidate and acknowledge their historical contributions to climate change, and rectify them. Climate reparations were a focus at the COP26 meeting held in the United Kingdom in 2021, with some representatives suggesting a goal of $100 billion per year of financial assistance by 2025 for climate-change adaptation in the most affected regions. Political leaders struck a deal to pay into such a fund at the COP27 summit held in Egypt in 2022, with the plan to iron out the details at COP28. It's promising, but critics suggest that the assistance is unlikely to pan out. Even if it does, they point out that the agreement's final text includes language that could be interpreted as approval of the continued use of natural gas, which is a bit like putting out a fire in the living room while fanning new flames in the bedroom.

There's also a case for climate reparations within nations. In the United States, where the ongoing legacies of slavery and genocide have exposed certain groups disproportionately to the impacts of climate change, these effects intersect with other forms of inequity. Neighborhoods with a higher proportion of low-income residents, immigrants, and non-European-Americans tend to have fewer trees, for instance, making children more vulnerable to the effects of extreme heat and other effects of climate change.

True sustainability isn't only about neutralizing carbon and other emissions, it's also about cultivating and sustaining health and justice for all, and for the Earth itself. Dr. Ayesha Khan, an infectious diseases scientist, grassroots organizer, writer, astrobiologist, and educator, has written that "the real problem isn't climate change, the problem is ecological destruction." As the creator of "abolitionist science," which takes a scientific approach to abolish systems of oppression, Khan warns against falling for the sheen of "green capitalism." Inequity, poverty, resource scarcity, overconsumption, and the destruction of habitats have not been sustainable. Capitalism and the synchronous global colonial pillaging of resources and destruction of habitats got us into this situation. Solutions rooted in capitalism won't get us out.

There are also nonchemical pollutants that interact with all of these other health-determining exposures that climate change compounds. Consider noise pollution, or unwanted sounds that persist in our environments. Dr. Erica Walker, an assistant professor of epidemiology at the Brown University School of Public Health, runs the Community Noise Lab, which holistically explores the relationship between community noise and health, largely through community research in Boston, Massachusetts, and in Mississippi. Noise pollution might seem harmless, but it has real impacts on children's health and disproportionately harms those in low-income neighborhoods that tend to be closer to roads and industrial facilities. "When people talk about noise, they kind of think about it as being like a first-world problem," Walker explains on a call in September 2022. There's this misconception that noise is "one of those things that you complain about because you have nothing else to complain about when the opposite is true." Children have "critical stages of development," so intense noise exposure over prolonged periods during these stages may lead to chronic or even long-term issues with cognitive function, learning, and more.

The accelerating impact of climate change also means that future generations will face even more severe exposure to its fallout. That's one reason why climate reparations don't only require a wealth transfer, but "a shift toward a more equitable and antiracist climate-change policy," write Manann Donoghoe and Andre M. Perry in a 2023 report for the Brookings Institution, a nonprofit research organization headquartered in Washington, DC. It requires not only reparations, they explain, but "a reparative stance" which "begins with granting reparations for Black Americans and advancing land reclamation for Native Americans" as a start, not only as a moral obligation but also to minimize climate-change impacts for the most vulnerable. It then goes beyond a transfer of wealth by aiming to dismantle structural determinants of inequity "that are likely to be amplified in emissions mitigation and climate-change adaptation policies" that haven't been intentionally designed to operate through an equity and antiracist lens.

One of the most fraught pieces surrounding equity and energy is that, while the activists, experts, and other sources I've spoken with over the years all agree that converting to renewable energy is imperative, there is often fierce disagreement about how to do that. I fear that this disagreement is derailing us.

Talking about nuclear energy raises hackles, and nuclear energy advocates still grapple with opposition despite saturating all major media outlets with messaging that suggests that nuclear energy is the best chance to save our planet. In the US, the Nuclear Energy Institute (NEI), a nuclear-industry trade association, argues that more nuclear plants will be a good thing because the electricity could make for greener cars: "It's not only about what kind of car we drive, but how we power our way of life. Nuclear energy makes sure that electric vehicles deliver their full potential as clean alternatives for the transportation sector."

Yes, powering electric vehicles with renewable energy is better than doing so with fossil fuels. But the NEI's statement and other similar rhetoric ignores the many problems associated with our current "way of life"—including massive, car-clogged highways and parking lots, unwalkable communities, and lack of public transit.

In an April 2020 blog post, the US Energy Department wrote, "When you hear the words 'clean energy,' what comes to mind? Most people immediately think of solar panels or wind turbines, but how many of you thought of nuclear energy? Nuclear is often left out of the 'clean energy' conversation." That the Green New

Deal may not have a place for nuclear energy has baffled proponents because the case for nuclear energy is so evidence-clad that it seems preposterous to oppose it.

They're not wrong. Nuclear energy is the most sustainable form of energy by several measures: it creates the smallest land footprint, the least waste, and the fewest emissions. Catastrophic events like the disaster in Chernobyl loom large, but the per capita risks of these disasters are exceedingly low. All sources of energy come with their own very real hazards. So one way to frame things is to look at which sources come with the lowest exposure to the least severe hazards.

Consider the body of data on the safety and benefits of our energy sources. In 2020, Hannah Ritchie, British data scientist and senior researcher at the University of Oxford in the Oxford Martin School, published a report on the cleanest and safest sources of energy for *Our World in Data*, for which she serves as deputy editor. "No energy source is completely safe," she writes in the introduction. "They all have short-term impacts on human health, either through air pollution or accidents. And they all have long-term impacts by contributing to climate change." When comparing energy sources, it can be helpful to think of safety in terms of the total number of human deaths per unit of electricity. The unit is the terawatt-hour (TWh), which, as Ritchie often points out, is about the same as the annual electricity consumption of 150,000 citizens in the European Union in 2021. This includes deaths from air pollution and accidents in the supply chain and is based on the assumption of 433 deaths from Chernobyl and 2,314 from Fukushima. By this measure, coal kills the most people by far—over 20 deaths per TWh. Oil comes in at a close second at around 18 deaths, followed by biomass (including wood, crops like corn, vegetable oils, manure, and sewage), with over 4 deaths, gas at less than 3 deaths, and hydropower at a little more than 1 death per TWh. Regarding hydropower, Ritchie points out that the death figure "is almost completely dominated by one event: the Banqiao Dam failure in China in 1975. It killed approximately 171,000 people. Otherwise, hydropower was very safe, with a death rate of just 0.04 deaths per TWh—comparable to nuclear, solar, and wind." These modern renewables have the lowest death rates by far, with wind at 0.04, nuclear at 0.03, and solar at 0.02 deaths per TWh.

That framing seems most useful when viewed within the context of legitimate concerns and distrust of technology with the potential for harm, concerns and distrust that stem from still-festering equity.

In the best-case scenario, nuclear power saves the day. This is the hope that led Heather Hoff and Kristin Zaitz, who both work at the Diablo Canyon Power Plant, the last remaining nuclear-power plant in the state of California, to found the non-profit Mothers for Nuclear, on Earth Day of 2016. They felt a responsibility to protect children and the planet they're set to inherit. Since then, the organization has built a global community of support for clean energy. For instance, on a 2023 phone call, Hoff points out that her state of California "has replaced a whole ton of imports and fossil fuel usage during the day with solar" which is "great." But to her, the push to close Diablo Canyon, and other nuclear plants around the world, is alarming. Nuclear energy makes most sense to her when she looks "across the spectrum of all of our values" including "protecting people's health, protecting the planet, minimizing [the use of] natural resources, and reliability of our energy supplies, because energy really does equal life and quality of life."

Hoff and Zaitz acknowledge that nuclear energy is far from perfect, but I can sense the urgency, and even the desperation, behind their enthusiasm. Both say they're not worried about their jobs, though they often get that question. "If Diablo Canyon is closed, the two of us will get other good jobs," they write. "But our kids will end up breathing dirtier air, and we will have failed to keep our promise to leave behind a world better than the one we inherited."

We could even source nuclear energy from existing bombs. It's happened before, through a US–Russia partnership spanning over twenty years beginning after the collapse of the Soviet Union. The equivalent of over 20,000 Soviet nukes were converted into zero-carbon energy. But the worst-case scenario of nuclear energy is a thing of our nightmares. As long as we keep control of the most hazardous processes in the uranium supply chain that fuels the nuclear-power life cycle, there's no reason to worry about the proliferation of nuclear weapons and war. But we can't know for sure that the peaceful use of nuclear fuel can always be maintained. There's a history of violation of Indigenous rights and lands in the greed for uranium, with the legacy of contaminated water and air still impacting Indigenous peoples.

Personally, I warily believe that supporting existing nuclear plants and adding more as part of the energy transition makes sense. I would like to see all fossil-fuel plants replaced by modern, renewable energy sources while ideally ensuring equity all around. Of course, that's far easier said than done. There are still a lot of unknowns and unachieved tasks ahead before we free ourselves from the reliance on fossil fuels. Energy-storage technologies have a way to go: to really use solar or wind to shift away from fossil fuels, we need systems that store those kinds of energy when the sun isn't shining and the wind isn't blowing. An equitable energy transition would center Indigenous peoples' rights and leadership, but so far, too many wind and solar projects have done the opposite.

It's worth noting that prioritizing or elevating the needs of selected nonhumans, including endangered species, while overlooking and subjugating certain groups of humans, has longed signaled injustice. More recently, I think of how the Madison city council unanimously banned the declawing of cats in 2021. Yes, it makes sense not to dismember our furry friends or to subject any creature to suffering. But this is the same city council that couldn't agree on banning chemical crowd-control agents that are highly harmful to humans. In this vein, white-centered environmentalists' agendas, with a focus on land conservation and nonhuman biodiversity protection without humans front and center, are laced with violence. Experts worldwide increasingly agree that, for biodiversity to thrive, conservation efforts must focus on humans as a primary component of a web of life and the conditions that sustain that web. Each thread depends on all of the others.

Progressive parents need to be aware of rampant *greenwashing*. The term has been around since the 1980s to describe misleading information suggesting that certain products, policies, or objectives are environmentally friendly. The problem is that greenwashed claims are ubiquitous, largely unregulated, and tricky to spot. Thinking of our doomed friend, the "this is fine" dog, an outsized focus on green choices for our individual families can be like throwing thimbles full of water on a raging fire.

Practically all large companies and institutions tout public climate strategies. These pledges, often with vague language and little regulatory oversight, make it increasingly challenging to recognize unsubstantiated green claims. There's nothing wrong with shopping at Whole Foods, wearing Patagonia, or using a so-called eco-friendly credit card, but these companies aren't here to put out the fire or fight injustice. As national campus campaign coordinator for the Environmental Justice and Climate Change Initiative Kari Fulton has said, high-end grocers like Whole Foods that claim to be green tend to avoid low-income communities, where people often end up "paying more for worse stuff" than families in more affluent communities.

With greenwashing, even the most harmful practices and products can exude an eco-friendly sheen. Writes Heglar, "If you thought oil companies were trafficking in outright climate denial or basking in the glow of right-wing delusion, you're in for a surprise." Oil companies present themselves as if they're "'just like us,' rolling up their sleeves and trying to find solutions to the climate crisis," but this "couldn't be further from the truth." The term *personal carbon footprint* was rolled out in 2000 in an award-winning campaign by the public relations firm Ogilvy on behalf of BP, Heglar points out.

In October 2019, in a continuation of the tried-and-true ad campaign, BP tweeted, "The first step to reducing your emissions is to know where you stand. Find out your #carbonfootprint with our new calculator & share your pledge today!" The company's calculator wasn't new in 2019, only updated. It's been around since 2004.

In Heglar's view, BP's tweet is a "textbook example" of greenwashing "where companies try to cover up their dirty work by making themselves appear more environmentally conscious than they are." This is the "same company that was champing at the bit to get at the oil in Iraq in the face of horrific human-rights violations. The same company that in 2019 alone saw more than $400 billion in profits," Heglar writes of BP's tweet. "*That* company was asking *us* about our carbon footprint. The nerve. The gall. The audacity. These people were playing right in my face." So instead of calculating her own carbon footprint, she replied to BP's tweet: "Bitch, what's yours???"

A newer poster child of greenwashing is the push to ditch plastic straws, which gained momentum in 2018 after a devastating photo of an endangered sea turtle with a plastic straw lodged in its nostril went viral. Plastic straws became a symbol of the scourge of single-use plastics, and soon, many establishments and communities were banning them. But as many of us have learned, ditching plastic straws does little to move the needle and is also a big drag for a lot of people. Disability-rights activists have pointed out that plastic straw bans have been a form of "eco-ableism," or discrimination against disabled people for the benefit of the environment and those who are able-bodied. **Bendy plastic straws have since served as a case study for the concept of universal design.** They help people with mobility, strength, or coordination issues, including children, drink and eat without spilling on themselves. Alternatives like paper straws that become mushy making them a choking hazard, metal straws that are sharp and lack the flexibility some people require to drink comfortably and safely, or silicone straws that are hard to clean and can harbor bacteria, are inferior. Ultimately, plastic straw bans have not only made life harder for people who need them, but they've also done little to save the Earth. **If there's a silver lining to the widespread opposition to plastic straws, some say it was that it got people talking about single-use plastics, like plastic bags, take-out containers and other food packaging, utensils, and water bottles. We know that plastics—a wide range of synthetic or semisynthetic materials derived from fossil-fuel-based chemicals that can be molded or melted into various shapes—are a problem.** Ingestion and exposure to various plastic debris, not just straws, harms many creatures, not just turtles. But eliminating items that make daily life equitable for humans isn't the solution. Think of grocery stores that stock precut fruits and veggies. Many decry the proliferation of prepared produce: *What's wrong with people nowadays that they can't even peel oranges and slice melons?!* Some scoff that prepared foods are more expensive and waste the plastic they often come packaged in. But the thing is, nothing has changed about people nowadays. There have always been folks who can't cut their own vegetables or peel their own oranges. Everyone has the right to a variety of nutritious food. I'm happy for those with the desire, bandwidth, time, and ability to buy, slice, and consume a whole melon. But the question is not what's wrong with people who buy precut produce or so-called convenience foods like prepared meals. The question is why people who need prepared food have to pay a price premium for a basic right. The question is how to ensure that everyone has access to good food while reducing harm to the planet.

Buying eco-friendly alternatives to plastics is often not a helpful solution, either. Claims like *biodegradable* and *compostable* on packaging are often "a big lie" says Daniela Ochoa Gonzalez, an advocate for environmental justice, composting, and clean air, and also an activist with Moms Clean Air Force, on a call in 2022. Composting is a crucial way to keep food scraps and nutrients out of landfills, she stresses, but outside of compostable food scraps and other specific types of organic waste, so-called compostable or biodegradable consumer products often don't break down, and when they do, they tend to break down into microplastics. Just because you can't see them doesn't mean they're not there.

What should parents do about plastic? Aluminum and most glass bottles and jars are considered "infinitely recyclable," so remove food debris and grease and recycle them. Otherwise, if you can't reuse something, *when in doubt, throw it out* in the trash and not the recycling bin, advises Kate O'Neill, a professor of environmental science, policy, and management at the University of California, Berkeley, on a call in September 2022. Her research on the global and local politics of wastes and recycling has led her to warn of the problems with "wishcycling," or "putting something in the recycling bin and hoping it will be recycled, even if there is little evidence to confirm this assumption." The term emerged in the mid-2010s with the increase of nonrecyclables contaminating the recycling stream. As responsible as it may feel to toss something into the recycling container, recycling requires someone to invest in turning it into another useful thing. Awareness of wishcycling as a concept started to spread in 2018 when China launched stringent restrictions on imports of most waste materials after having purchased millions of tons of it from wealthy nations over the preceding twenty years or so. The restrictions created massive waste backups in the US and other wealthy nations where governments had failed to create their own robust recycling systems. This has led to pileups of stuff that people thought they were recycling ending up in landfills instead.

O'Neill calls recycling in the US an "industry" that was launched in the 1970s in response to public concern over litter and waste. Recycling programs helped waste to not "seem entirely bad if it could lead to the creation of new products." Prorecycling messaging, including resin identification codes inside the now-familiar triangle of chasing arrows found on plastics began to imply that items with a triangle are recyclable, "even though that was usually far from the truth," write O'Neill and coauthor Jessica Heiges in a 2022 article in *The Conversation*. They explain that only resins labeled #1 (polyethylene terephthalate, or PET) and #2 (high-density polyethylene, or HDPE) are relatively easy to recycle and have viable markets. A lot of what ends up in recycling doesn't actually get recycled. Though there are recycling programs for plastic shopping bags, for instance, which can be turned into things like plastic park benches, most end up in landfills, the environment, and oceans, or contaminating the recycling stream. Instead of wishful thinking, it's worth checking your municipality's recycling guidelines.

It makes sense to avoid single-use plastics if and whenever you can and, at the same time, avoid expressing judgment of people for using them. I hope that my children will never assume to know another person's circumstance or reason for consuming a specific product, let alone judge them for it. Some of us may be conditioned to condemn others' choices, but I believe that teaching our children to keep it to themselves is teaching an example of kindness. We are not the consumption police. This problem is far bigger than our own personal choices. As O'Neill and Heiges put it, "the global waste crisis wasn't created by consumers who failed to wash mayonnaise jars or separate out plastic bags." The biggest drivers include capitalistic reliance on consumption, a lack of standardized recycling policies, and the devaluation of used resources.

As much as I worry about the outsized burden on individuals to solve largely systemic problems, as individual parents we can still make a difference. Yes, we need to keep pressure on corporations to cut emissions and stop the destruction. But that doesn't mean that parents should give up on making impactful individual choices. At the very least, some experts believe that widespread individual action can spur political, systemic change through a shift in societal beliefs and values. But it could do more than that. It could help keep us from breaching that terrible threshold.

"Yes, you should still reduce your personal carbon footprint," writes Jenny Splitter in a September 2022 newsletter. Some individual actions are important and even critical for slowing the effects of climate change. Evidence suggests that, together, our household choices have the potential to produce up to roughly 25–30% of the total emissions reductions needed to avoid dangerous climate change of 1.5°C. "[I]n their urgency to generate much-needed collective action, some climate advocates may be inadvertently discouraging the kinds of behavioral change that we actually do need to be making."

Again, let's look at food.

Even though emissions from agriculture are the second highest after the energy sector, they "continue to be downplayed or misrepresented." Splitter says that one big misconception is that eating locally grown food makes the biggest difference. In reality, while eating locally grown food can be great for supporting your community and local farmers, it's not necessarily better for the environment. Because the transportation sector overall is a massive emissions source, "it's easy to assume" that transportation accounts for a major part of food-systems emissions, but overall, its contribution is a very small percentage of them.

On the whole, most food-related emissions come from the

farming and production, and not the transportation, of food. That's why experts say that what you eat matters a lot more than how far it traveled to reach you. Local beef almost certainly has a higher carbon footprint than lentils sourced from anywhere on Earth. Air-freighted food does have relatively high transport emissions, though. Not much of our food is air freighted except for those that need to be consumed shortly after harvest; for instance, asparagus and berries are commonly transported by air. By contrast, fruits and veggies with a longer shelf life, like apples, cabbages, and carrots, have lower transportation emissions because they tend to get to us by boat, truck, or rail. Frozen fruits or veggies are also not typically air freighted because there isn't a big rush to get them to consumers.

It is often hard to identify foods that have traveled by air because they're rarely labeled as such. This makes them difficult to avoid. If you want to try, it can help to avoid fresh foods that have a very short shelf life and have traveled a long way (country-of-origin labels can help with this). This especially tends to be true for foods where there is a strong emphasis on freshness: for these products, transport speed is a priority.

So if you want to reduce the carbon footprint of your diet, avoid the most commonly air-freighted foods where you can. But more importantly, you can make a larger difference by focusing on what you eat than eating local. Eating less meat and dairy will reduce your footprint by much more than buying local.

At the same time, it can make sense to buy local to support your community. And since justice matters just as much as emissions, it also makes sense to think of the impacts of foods that that aren't locally sourced. Daniela Ochoa Gonzalez asks me to consider progressive parents who purchase avocados—more are grown in her home state of Michoacán in Mexico than anywhere else in the world, largely for export—because they "think that they're nourishing their children" with the fruit's purported health benefits. Compared to several other problematic crops and food products that are known to harm local environments and communities where they're grown and produced, like chocolate and palm oil, avocados are particularly notorious for going bad in the blink of an eye after people bring them home. Having seen firsthand the tragic effects on the environment and people in her home state, the stark increase in consumption of avocados in the US since the late 1990s, and moreover the amount that end up uneaten in the garbage, is hard to accept for Gonzalez.

Avocado farming tends to use more water than even almonds—which are known as a particularly thirsty crop—driving devastating water scarcity, deforestation, pollution and depletion of soil nutrients. There is also targeted violence from drug cartels that seek to control the industry and sometimes demand protection money from farmers. Researchers have estimated that rapid deforestation and increasing reliance on pesticides has harmed local flora and fauna, including monarch butterflies. As avocados deplete the nutrient-rich soil, farmers must turn to industrial chemical fertilizers, which are dangerously scarce globally. Some of the agricultural chemicals used for avocado farming contaminate the subsoil and leach into waterways. Officials say that even though a consumer boycott of avocados might seem like the obvious answer, especially since avocados are increasingly known as "the blood diamonds of Mexico," a sudden slump in demand could be disastrous for the local economy. Cutting down on avocado consumption and avoiding avocado waste seems like a worthwhile start for individual families. When someone does buy an avocado, it makes sense to be vigilant about consuming it before it goes overripe and composting the skin and seed.

Most agricultural GHG emissions come from methane released in cattle belches, as Splitter often points out, and from land use by humans for various purposes. Some also come from the massive stream of manure from these animals. Addressing climate change depends largely on how we use our land because it has a huge impact on carbon sources and sinks.

Humans have been shaping the land and life on Earth for thousands of years. Today, agriculture occupies roughly 40 percent of the Earth's ice-free surface. On the whole, animal agriculture is the least efficient type of farming in terms of land, with all of the land required to produce beef—including pastureland and feed-crop land—occupying around a hundred times more space than plant crops grown for human consumption.

Studies show that eating less meat and wasting less food are two of the most powerful individual actions to reduce climate emissions. According to the World Resources Institute, which used data from 2016 to come up with a scorecard of GHG emissions per gram of protein for various foods, wheat, corn, beans, chickpeas, and lentils have the lowest emissions, while beef, lamb, and goat have the highest, even if they're grass-fed. Poultry, pork, and dairy fall in between.

It doesn't have to be all-or-nothing. People can make a difference by cutting back on their family's intake to the equivalent of around 1.5 or fewer beef burgers per person per week. To reduce food waste, Splitter suggests menu planning, being more mindful about how much we buy at the store and order from a restaurant, and using items past their sell-by dates.

In the US, best-if-used-by dates indicate when a product will have the best flavor or quality, and sell-by dates indicate how long to display the product for sale. These aren't safety dates. "In an effort to reduce food waste, it is important that consumers understand that the dates applied to food are for quality and not for safety," says the USDA. "Food products are safe to consume past the date on the label, and regardless of the date, consumers should evaluate the quality of the food product prior to its consumption."

Popular vegan protein-rich foods and meat alternatives are fine options. Tofu, seitan, and processed plant-based products account for far lower emissions by and large than animal meat. At the same time, Khan warns that only considering CO_2 emissions of what we eat is oversimplifying. Consider that American global food conglomerate Cargill has emerged as a leader in the plant-based meat industry in the 2020s, and many of these products are made using soy and corn, both of which are crops that contribute to ecological damage. Alternative meats "will be a tool to further stratify populations across the globe and continue to separate humans from the ecosystems around us." I understand Khan's concern—replacing traditional foods with mass-produced plant-based protein foods lines the pockets of industries and their executives and may contribute to the power imbalances embedded in the food system. I hold this complexity in my heart whenever I eat a meat alternative or feed one to my kids, which, frankly, I do fairly regularly.

What about milk? Reports have suggested that almond milk is terrible for the environment, especially in California where many of the almonds used to produce it can exacerbate drought conditions. Several of my peers avoid almond milk for this reason. I use almond milk every day. "Every bite of food we eat comes at a cost, whether you measure that cost in methane emitted from cow burps, herbicides used to save soybeans from weeds, or hours worked by farm laborers to pick and process food," writes Splitter in a *SciMoms* post. Some foods come with a higher environmental cost than others.

Environmental costs of food can be broken down into components including emissions, land use, and water use. Compared with plant-based milk, the evidence shows that dairy milk requires more land and water to produce than almond milk and emits more GHGs. One reason that beef and dairy-milk products generate such high GHG emissions is because of the way cows, as ruminant animals with four stomach compartments, including one called the rumen, digest their food. The rumen ferments its contents, breaking down tough feed like hay that humans wouldn't want to ingest. This fermentation process leads these animals to release around 40% of the global methane measured on an annual basis, again, mostly in the form of belches. Methane is a far more potent greenhouse gas than carbon—more than twenty-five times more potent at trapping heat in the atmosphere. The second big reason that dairy milk has a high-emissions cost is because of the land required to raise and feed dairy cows. It takes a lot more land to raise dairy cows than it does to grow almonds, oats, rice, or coconuts for milk.

Cooking also contributes to emissions, and lately, gas appliances, especially stoves, and the neighborhood pipelines that supply them, have increasingly been in the news for their release of methane. One 2022 study found that the amount of this potent GHG released by gas stoves every year is comparable in climate impact to the annual CO2 emissions of around half a million cars. The compounds that gas stoves release are also known to harm human health, including the developing lungs and brains of children. In cities like Boston, there are zones and areas of neglect, says Nathan Phillips, a professor at Boston University, who studies land-climate interactions in terrestrial ecosystems and human-dominated environments. "Homes that cook with gas, including stoves that aren't well-maintained, are disproportionately located in lower-income communities," he tells me on a 2022 call. So are poorly maintained pipelines that leak outdoors. In addition to contributing to poor air quality and harming human health, these leaks also kill trees, and "those trees don't get replaced or reported," contributing to the formation of "urban heat islands at the micro level, at the neighborhood level."

System-level changes to phase out the use of natural gas in homes and neighborhoods are happening slowly, but individuals can make a difference in the meantime, says Phillips. For those with a gas stove, there's no need to spring for a pricey replacement. He quips that for stovetops, "the price of admission to our great energy transition is fifty bucks," which was the approximate price in USD of the portable induction cooktop that he and his family primarily use for their cooking. Electric air fryers, toaster ovens, and electric kettles for hot water can also be useful components of a family's "cooking toolkit." He encourages parents to not take actions like switching to electric appliances "in isolation" but to share them with neighbors and friends. Phillips believes that this is "how we build our communities and build system change," while also doing our best to "go straight to the top and pressure our elected officials to get the policies in place at every level," including reducing reliance on fossil fuels to generate electricity.

One way to begin connecting these individual actions into collective action, from reducing meat in our diets to reducing the use of gas cooktops, is to talk about it, Splitter says. It's harder than it sounds because food is personal. "No one has deep attachments to their light bulbs or family traditions that center around water heaters," she quips. "Yet start talking about even just the use of a gas cooktop and, whoo boy, you will get some serious pushback" and "that's before we even get to what's on the plate."

We know that some people consume meat and dairy for cultural and personal reasons. Some nations and groups have historically been deprived of hunting and consuming traditional high-protein components of their diets, while some nations and groups have consumed far more than their share for generations. I don't judge others for their consumption of any specific foods, including meat. I'm also impressed with those who adapt their own favorite foods, including the ones passed down from generation to generation, with substitutes for meat and dairy. If everyone who already makes these small shifts at home in turn talks to their friends and family about eating less beef each week, "perhaps that can begin to add up to meaningful change," Splitter says.

I'm skeptical when the consumption of new goods is touted as a solution, even when those goods are made with postconsumer recycled material. For necessary items, it makes sense to seek out recycled or recyclable materials, where possible. My kids and I own a few products that are proudly made with recycled plastic—including shoes and clothing—but do I need them, and did these purchases really help the environment? Doubtful. There's also been increasing attention to the invisible plastic fibers that leach from synthetic clothing into wastewater when washed. Thrifting is one alternative and a necessary part of some people's lives, but it isn't a solution to the harms of excess consumption, either. It seems counterintuitive, but in terms of the energy required for transportation and the associated emissions, shopping online with delivery—for new or used items—can be as green or greener in terms of emissions than shopping at a local brick-and-mortar store. As journalist Tim Heffernan put it in *Wirecutter* in 2021, "One van delivering 50 packages is much more efficient than 50 people driving to the store." But if someone is driving to multiple stores to search for an item and ultimately choosing to make their purchase online, then that purchase wasn't particularly environmentally friendly. Some research also suggests that online shopping can be more efficient when people are able to opt for longer delivery times. Still, among other concerns about online shopping, I worry about the delivery drivers and other workers with the worsening heat waves and no federal law requiring that delivery vehicles have air conditioning.

Outside of food, whenever possible, it doesn't hurt to strive to consume less with the understanding that it won't solve all of our problems and that minimalism is not accessible to everyone. When our family requires something that doesn't need to be brand-new, we often get it from online local marketplaces, buy-nothing groups, secondhand stores, or community members who no longer have use for an item. We try to buy only what we need, though the distinction between wants and needs can be hazy.

Another part of consuming less is how we get around. Of that 25–30% of estimated emissions that individuals might collectively reduce, travel is another big category that we can control, including the use of public transit.

As for what kind of car parents should drive, if you live in a place where public transit is inconvenient and you're replacing your old car, buying electric will generally give you a lower carbon footprint than buying a gas-powered vehicle. But ideally, communities everywhere will prioritize public transit, says Dr. Kari Watkins, an associate professor in civil and environmental engineering at the University of California, Davis who studies ways to make the transportation system easier to use, more sustainable, healthier, and more efficient. On an individual level, switching from a nonelectric vehicle to an EV "is going to have a little bit of an environmental impact, so that's a great place to start." But to be as sustainable as possible, "we need to electrify the transit fleet itself."

One way to measure emissions is per-passenger mile (or kilometer) or trip. National averages demonstrate that public transportation produces significantly lower greenhouse gas emissions per-passenger mile than private vehicles. The fewer empty seats on a bus or train, the lower the per-passenger emissions.

For those who can swing it, "using transit goes a step beyond" just your own personal carbon footprint because, "by you paying that fare, you're allowing that service to exist for other people who need that service as well. I think it's also a really great way for your kids to understand the community around them and not be isolated from that community." Watkins points out that switching to individually owned EVs "is not going to help congestion, it's not going to help the safety picture" for pedestrians and passengers. And it's not going to help that urban sprawl—a measure of the expansion of cities into suburbs and other low-density development—coupled with inconvenient public transit can add precious time to commutes.

Inequity thrives wherever driving a car is far less of a hassle than taking public transit. The connection between the lack of convenient public transit and health disparities is undeniable. Since public transit generally takes much longer than driving somewhere, there's "this barrier to taking trips, where you're only going to take the trips that you have to take," explains Watkins. "You have to pay the bills, so you're going to get yourself to work," but anything that isn't "entirely absolutely necessary, you're not going to do because there's such a barrier in trying to get there." In this way, someone might get their kids to the doctor because people are trying to make sure their kids thrive. But "are they going to get themselves to the doctor for preventative care? Probably not." If someone has to take "one bus connecting to another in order to get," say, a vaccine, "it takes an awful lot to decide that that's something that you're going to do." She asks parents who drive a car to "think about every trip you make on a day-to-day basis." If you're dependent on transit, "there's a lot that is going to very quickly fall off of that list," of errands. As for the carbon footprint associated with air travel, it helps to take fewer flights overall and to try to make our flights more worthwhile, Watkins advises. Try to stay near a destination for longer.

Though I'm not worried about glyphosate in children's hummus and toasted oats specifically, I do worry about the problems associated with some of the crops that it's widely used on. Field corn, cotton, and soy, the majority of which has been genetically engineered to tolerate it, dominate global agriculture, and together, their harm to children is huge, albeit indirect. Let's zoom in on corn—not sweet corn (you know, the corn that changes everything when you try it with butter) but field corn. **Corn isn't just a crop, it's a core piece of an industrial complex with tendrils that touch everything that affects children's wellbeing, from how our land is used to the food we eat to how we get around.** America's single biggest, most heavily subsidized crop in 2019, field corn is widely considered the lifeblood of the Midwest. The majority of this crop feeds animals raised for human consumption and fuels cars in the form of ethanol. It's also used in everything from plastics marketed as biodegradable to carpeting and textiles. Only a small amount of field corn is ingested by humans in food, in the form of high-fructose corn syrup, other sweeteners, and cereals.

To say that corn is ubiquitous would be an understatement. As a blogger for the Texas Farm Bureau put it, "from the moment you wake up in the morning to the time you lie down at night, corn is in your life. It could be in your bedding, carpet, fuel, soda, beef, crayons, plastic, and more." No matter where you are, "know that part of your day was brought to you by American corn farmers."

Corn can seem like an environmental boon. As the USDA communications office put it in a 2015 fact sheet, "corn yields per acre are 8 times more than they were a century ago, ensuring US corn supplies keep up with growing global demand." Ethanol, for instance, is marketed as much cleaner than gasoline: a 2020 analysis found that using corn-based ethanol in place of gasoline reduces life-cycle GHG emissions on average by 40%. Viewed through other lenses, corn is an environmental and health disaster. Those narratives have been competing for decades, and it's hard to see any winners.

To some degree, genetic modification has helped increase corn yields. The genetically engineered traits of insect resistance and herbicide tolerance are thought to have contributed in part to the rise in production per unit of land. As part of a toolbox of useful plant breeding methods, agricultural genetic engineering is capable of elegant feats, like creating plant varieties that are resistant to diseases that can wipe out crops. But the regulatory landscape has largely relegated genetic engineering technologies to commodity crops that benefit producers and contribute to ecological demise.

No, it's not genetic modification itself that worries me, nor is glyphosate in my kids' breakfast. What worries me is that our food system has been dominated by problematic crops since well before genetic modification and Roundup existed.

Silvia Secchi, a professor of geographical and sustainability sciences at the University of Iowa, studies the environmental impacts of agricultural land use, particularly water quality and carbon, and the interplay between agricultural, conservation, and energy policies in the region. There is "a massive amount of greenwashing" that keeps everyone "making the choices that we've been making, and makes them appear sustainable," she tells me on a call in May of 2022. But even though ethanol releases fewer emissions than gasoline, its impact on water pollution, which proponents brush over, is not pretty.

Despite mounting pressure to improve public transportation, cars reign supreme, with ethanol fueling the expansion of highways and roads. Our production system has "focused on some of these commodity crops and associated livestock production systems," says Secchi. "Because the main uses of corn are for ethanol and for feed," we've essentially "created a system over decades that rewards that type of production," she explains. "It's almost like we produce all this corn so we need to find uses for it." It's really a "vicious circle" in which we produce more, so then "we have to find more uses" for it, and then "we get more technology to produce even more," which increasingly locks us "into the circle."

Secchi vents that there aren't sufficient "mandatory changes" required of industries. "We don't force anybody to do things that they don't want to do," and on top of that, there "is an overreliance on technological fixes." There's this idea that we can simply "switch the way we drive from internal-combustion engine cars to electric cars, but we don't fundamentally change" things like "the character of our neighborhoods, or we don't massively increase the availability of public transportation." Ultimately, "we're making changes that are not the size that they need to be to truly address climate change, but we feel like we've done enough. So we are absolved, and we don't have to do anything else." She's particularly concerned that "this approach disproportionately affects poor people, particularly poor people in the global south" who can't simply switch to electric vehicles. She warns against losing focus of the big picture, which is that "our water system is connected to our energy system and it's connected to our food system."

Ultimately, we're left with a higher-tech, twenty-first-century version of the old-school status quo in agriculture, like the marginal benefits that biotechnology has brought to crops that already dominated American farmland over the past century—crops that hearken back to yesteryear and to the conservative yearning for American greatness.

"There was no reason to let it last this long and get this bad," as KC Green's comic dog put it. "This is not fine."

8

vaccines

Vaccines are among the most lifesaving medical advance-ments ever. All recommended vaccines are hugely beneficial and pose an extremely low risk to the vast majority of people. Vaccines save millions of lives every year. These are the facts.

Vaccines are not perfect. On an individual level, vaccines ideally equip our immune systems with the information to build up a specific arsenal, army, and strategy to protect us against a particular viral or bacterial invasion. There are vaccines that protect against more than thirty diseases and counting, though not all of these are given routinely. On a community level, if a high-enough percentage of a population has immunity against a disease, the more protected the group is as a whole, and the safer it is for the most vulnerable people in the group, including babies who are too young to receive certain vaccines, those with chronic health conditions, and people with contraindications to certain vaccines, including those who are severely immuno-compromised. This group protection is called herd immunity, or community immunity. In some ways, vaccination is like voting: it's not always ideal, and the system is flawed, but it's one of a few actions that can make a difference, and even save lives.

The eradication of smallpox and the near-eradication of polio are two of vaccinations' biggest success stories. But every pathogen behaves differently, which means that every vaccine needs to be developed to do the unique job of inducing protection against each one. In a perfect world, all vaccines would eventually eradicate the disease they protect against. Some experts believe that eradication is possible with measles, but the failure of systems to prioritize measles eradication, combined with pockets of unvaccinated folks, has led to continued outbreaks of the illness that causes high fever, severe cough, and a telltale rash. It was practically an inevitable rite of childhood, causing an estimated 2.6 million deaths each year prior to the introduction of vaccination worldwide in 1963. The measles shot is highly effective, meaning that it is pretty adept at training our immune systems to spot this virus and kick it to the curb. It's a two-and-done deal; nearly all children who receive the recommended two doses of the measles, mumps, and rubella, or MMR, vaccine are considered to be immune against measles for life, though some research suggests that immunity from this vaccine may eventually start to wane. A handful of other vaccines, including those for HPV and hepatitis B, are also thought to be particularly good at providing long-term immunity to nearly all who receive the recommended series of doses. That's in large part because these pathogens aren't very good at mutating, and because these vaccines are good at triggering long-term, sustained immune-system defenses, largely in the form of antibodies that can remember, spot, and disable their distinct targets. These vaccines come closest to preventing both disease and transmission of the illness they protect against.

Other vaccines have a harder task because some pathogens are trickier than others. For instance, the proteins on the surface of the influenza virus that help it infect cells—and that antibodies and immune cells can recognize and target—change relatively often, which is why there's a new shot annually. For some diseases, people need another dose of the same vaccine every so often to rev their immune system's vigilance, which can get sluggish over time. Not all vaccines prevent transmission, but they all protect against severe illness, hospitalization, and death in most of the vaccinated population. The more of the population that is vaccinated, the better these vaccines work to protect everyone. Herd immunity helps some infectious diseases stay contained enough for health systems to handle. Herd immunity can dwindle in some pockets of the population, due to a decrease in vaccination, waning immunity from previous vaccines or illnesses, and other factors, causing outbreaks that are serious enough to stress local health systems and take a toll on everyone. **All in all, every recommended vaccine is known to protect against the worst outcomes of their respective illnesses and save lives. Vaccines are not a panacea. They're amazing, and I'm thankful for them. But they're only one of multiple layers of protection for communities. Like anything else in the world, no vaccine is risk-free, but for the vast majority of people, the risks of vaccinating are vanishingly low while the risks of contracting one of these diseases without the protection from a vaccine are high.**

Some can't help but blame parents who don't vaccinate their children for the resurgence of diseases like measles and for the slow burn of COVID-19. But as tempting as it may be to point the finger at parents of unvaccinated kids, those who deserve the bulk of our ire are the systems that shape the trajectory of diseases and perpetuate global inequity in vaccine distribution and other resources not only for COVID-19 but other illnesses, too. Anti-vaccine leaders are abhorrent, but so was the CDC for dropping crucial layers of protection like indoor masking in the first half of 2021. In May of 2023, the CDC officially ended the COVID-19 public-health emergency, not because the pandemic is over but in large part because tracking COVID cases is taxing to an already overburdened health system. Experts stress that the virus is still very much with us, and, to protect the most vulnerable, we will likely require more vaccination and masking down the line.

With the help of the internet, anti-vaccine sentiment surged starting in the late 1990s following the publishing of the infamous series of retracted papers linking the MMR vaccine with autism by the now-disgraced former gastroenterologist Andrew Wakefield and his colleagues—which subsequently fanned the flames of ableism against neurodivergent children and adults. Vaccines have never caused autism. Over the years, vaccine hesitation has gotten so bad that in 2019 the WHO declared it one of the top ten threats to global health.

Tara C. Smith, PhD, a professor at the Kent State University College of Public Health who studies zoonotic infections and also writes extensively about vaccine hesitancy, often describes what she has called the "cast of characters" who are influential and play a role in perpetuating vaccine misinformation. "Although many parents may repeat uncritically the information they receive from vaccine-denial groups, these claims rarely originate with the parent de novo," she explains in a 2017 review article on vaccine rejection and hesitancy. The media and internet are rife with vaccine myths that are "circulated by a variety of influential individuals and organizations and are read and repeated by parents and other media consumers." These individuals have included model, actor, and television personality Jenny McCarthy, celebrity doctor Mehmet Oz, Robert F. Kennedy Jr., and others. Then there are social-media and parenting-group anti-vaccine bullies, who go as far as accusing parents whose children have died from vaccine-preventable illnesses of lying.

While the internet has provided vaccine opposition with a

larger venue, anti-vaccination attitudes have existed for as long as there have been vaccines.

Old-timey pamphlets reveal that some people have always distrusted scientists and doctors and that some parents have always hesitated or refused to vaccinate their children. In all likelihood, these attitudes existed *before* modern vaccines. Records as early as the eighteenth century show that people in parts of Asia and Africa developed and were practicing earlier forms of inoculation, called variolation, against smallpox, including scratching pus into healthy children's skin and blowing powdered smallpox scabs into healthy people's noses. These rudimentary forms of inoculation were far less safe than modern vaccines, but they were so effective that, eventually, the practice spread to Europe and the Americas. The risk of death from variolation was around 1%, which is pretty high, but far lower than the mortality rate of catching smallpox, which happened to nearly everyone and killed about one in three infected, so as proponents saw it, the benefits outweighed the risks. Records also suggest that while many lined up for variolation procedures, others opposed it staunchly. I would be shocked if the practice didn't utterly appall and terrify some parents and set one clique against another.

Some anti-vaccine misinformation and disinformation has always seemed downright tinfoil-hat ridiculous, like the belief that COVID vaccines are a government ploy to inject microchips into recipients, or even that Bill Gates created the pandemic with the plan to do so. But people also have legitimate concerns about vaccines stemming from the very first immunizations that were tested on enslaved people, orphaned children, and prisoners. Lumping these concerns about vaccines together with unsubstantiated conspiracy theories doesn't make sense. The themes that underlie anti-vaccine sentiment have remained more or less consistent for centuries, including that Big Pharma is exploitative and profit-driven, that the chemicals in vaccines are harmful, that natural immunity is better, and that we can't trust our government to protect us.

Yes, the pharmaceutical industry is highly predatory and our government is hardly a beacon of trustworthiness. Anxiety around pharmaceutical interventions is understandable, especially when we're injecting them into our kids' bodies, but there are better ways to channel justified distrust of the system than avoiding vaccines. As a progressive parent with a healthy distrust of the government and of the institution of medicine, one thing I do trust is the CDC-recommended vaccine schedule for children and adults.

There is nothing wrong with having questions or hesitation about vaccines. There's a lot more variability than just the pro- versus anti-vaccine dichotomy. Some people strongly support vaccinations, or are what we might think of as pro-vaccine. Others support vaccination but have concerns, some are the watch-and-wait types who eventually come around, and some may also distrust the system; we can think of all of them as vaccine-hesitant. For some, it may be inconvenient to receive vaccines. Not as many people are straight-up anti-vax as it might seem.

While it's undoubtedly crucial to refute myths about vaccines, it makes sense to turn our frustration against the system. Though public-health messaging often tries to garner trust, placing the onus largely on individuals to have trust in vaccination may be misguided. For one, this framing ignores that many people can and do end up choosing to get vaccinated even while they feel distrust or fear. This fear doesn't make them stupid, and getting vaccinated despite that fear is brave. As soothing as it might be for vaccine enthusiasts to believe that the world would be a far better place if more people would just believe in vaccines, that idea hasn't been putting out the bulk of the fires of disease.

As Victor Lopez-Carmen has pointed out, native life expectancy in the US dropped more than any other group during the pandemic despite having the highest vaccination rates. The fact that native-led vaccination campaigns have "saved so many lives, but that systemic racism and its health impacts" are still killing people makes it clear that "vaccinations only go so far." Lopez-Carmen says that there's a white, classist narrative that vaccination will protect everyone equally, but that's not the case. He finds it unsettling that "there's a normativity to messaging" that "totally ignores" that marginalized communities have higher rates of comorbidities that can lead to complications.

There are other ways that the systemic urge to demand trust from the public is misguided. With increasing attention to the legacy of racism in the United States, the discourse around the COVID-19 vaccine has also turned its focus to distrust of vaccines in Black communities. But some experts argue that this framing is skewed: "[A]ssertions that patient mistrust drives disparities" in vaccination obscure the real causes of racial health inequities and "tacitly blames affected patients for their disproportionate suffering." Some US doctors chalk up distrust of the medical system by Black and other people of color, including distrust of vaccines, to three key historical atrocities: 1) the so-called father of gynecology J. Marion Sims's experimentation on enslaved Black women; 2) the development of the first human cell line from Henrietta Lacks's tumor biopsy without her consent in the 1950s; and 3) the infamous Tuskegee syphilis study that began in 1932, in which researchers exploited their Black research subjects for forty years and withheld the information that a treatment became available in 1947. In Sims's papers, he only mentioned three of the exploited subjects, who had no say in their excruciating torture, by name: Anarcha, who was a teenager—a child—and Betsy, and Lucy. The implication is that Black people who distrust the medical system, including vaccines, are irrational in holding on to grievances from long ago. Reducing Black people's distrust of medicine to just Sims, Lacks, and Tuskegee falsely relegates racial injustice in medicine to the past.

As two MDs writing in the *New England Journal of Medicine* put it, "[e]very day, Black Americans have their pain denied, their conditions misdiagnosed, and necessary treatment withheld by physicians. In these moments, those patients are probably not historicizing their frustration by recalling Tuskegee, but rather contemplating how an institution sworn to do no harm has failed them." The authors point out that infant mortality is halved when Black newborns are cared for by Black rather than white physicians. Babies have not had the opportunity to learn American history. The fact that the race of an infant's doctor can predict the likelihood of life or death shows us why distrust is not the result of historical atrocities. It's the result of present injustice. Infants "cannot contemplate historical traumas: they can still experience everyday racism and disrespect."

An outsized focus on vaccine opposition leads to misrepresentations about and scapegoating of unvaccinated people. Analyses of the internet discourse have suggested increased polarization between pro- and anti-vaccine segments. For instance, a 2017 article at the Wellcome Collection explains that "[m]any of the memes circulated in response to anti-vaccination arguments make identity-based attacks. It's common to question the intelligence or education" of the anti-vaccine target. "The implied logic of this is clear: anti-vaxxers are unable to understand the evidence in favor of vaccines—it's too difficult for them—and if they could understand it, they would change their positions. The simplicity of this theory is attractive and suggests an easy solution to vaccine refusal, but unfortunately it's false."

Also, while it can be helpful to provide missing information to reassure fellow parents, Smith and other experts on vaccine hesitation and denial warn against the impulse to fall into the "information deficit model" of communication, which assumes that the public is merely uneducated or undereducated about vaccines, and that providing additional factual information will fill this knowledge gap and lead people toward vaccinating. One of the biggest mistakes someone can make as a pro-vaccine parent talking to another mom or dad on the playground is to "assume you know anything about why someone may not be vaccinating" says Smith.

Even public-health officials have wrongly blamed the drawn-out COVID-19 pandemic on the unvaccinated specifically, including CDC director Rochelle Walensky who decried it as a "pandemic of the unvaccinated" in 2021.

Yet again, some officials have blamed the fallout of this pandemic disproportionately on the choices of individuals instead of on the failures of the system. "The current US approach continues to undermine the fundamental notion that all people are equal in dignity and rights," write the authors of a 2021 commentary in the journal *eClinicalMedicine*, published by *The Lancet*. This approach "implicitly assumes that those who become ill are responsible for their own suffering and that their deaths are acceptable—because they could have been vaccinated. These moral deficiencies reflect a larger neglect of collective responsibility, equity, and human rights in US public-health policy."

It would be great to see more COVID-19 vaccination in the United States and vaccine equity globally. Unvaccinated children and adults are still dying of COVID, many more are suffering from long-term effects from it, and countless others will face health consequences years down the road. The good news is that the number of people vaccinated against it is increasing. At the same time, vaccinated people are also catching and spreading this illness, and the most vulnerable pay the steepest price.

Yet again, outside of pushing systems to ensure true justice in public health for all, there are a few things individual parents can do and even a few ways to potentially help someone with doubts about vaccines think through them, even if that someone is yourself or a loved one.

First, it's worth becoming familiar with some of the most common concerns that lead to vaccine hesitancy.

One is that kids are receiving "too many vaccines too soon." The current vaccine schedule, in which children receive vaccines regularly starting at birth, can seem overwhelming, so some parents think it may be beneficial to follow an alternative schedule that spaces out immunizations. It's true that kids get more shots nowadays than my fellow millennials did when we were little.

"Children get more shots today simply because there are more vaccines," says fellow SciParent Layla Katiraee. Shots for hepatitis B didn't exist when she was born and neither did vaccination for chicken pox. Children today are "protected against even more diseases" than many of us were when we were kids. She wants people to consider how awesome it is that there's now a shot that can help prevent a type of cancer. Again, we have our problems with the CDC, but the vaccination schedule isn't one. That's why we urge our friends and loved ones to stick to the CDC's recommended schedule or their country's equivalent. Choosing a delayed schedule unnecessarily increases risks.

The Advisory Committee on Immunization Practices (ACIP), a committee of fifteen voting members within the CDC, is responsible for developing vaccine recommendations for the civilian population in the US. The Secretary of the US Department of Health and Human Services selects these members following a nomination or application process. Fourteen of the members have expertise in vaccinology, immunology, pediatrics, internal medicine, nursing, family medicine, virology, public health, infectious diseases, and/or preventive medicine, and one member is a consumer representative who provides perspectives on the social and community aspects of vaccination. ACIP also includes eight ex officio members who represent other federal agencies with responsibility for immunization programs in the United States, and thirty nonvoting representatives of liaison organizations that bring related immunization expertise.

The committee generally meets three times a year to review

the latest research and data for each vaccine. It creates a schedule to provide maximum protection, as early as possible, without problematic interactions between different vaccines. The information ACIP reviews includes the severity of the disease and the potential for causing long-term health problems or death. They also consider the number of children who get the disease if there is no vaccine. Vaccines that do not provide benefits to many children may not be recommended as part of the routine schedule.

By contrast, alternate schedules "are completely made up," says Katiraee. "They are arbitrary, untested, not evaluated by experts, and not subject to any scrutiny," and "choosing an untested schedule over a tested schedule" exposes children to unnecessary and preventable risks.

Another common question is whether a vaccine can give someone the disease it's supposed to prevent. The answer is technically *yes* for specific vaccines, but incredibly rarely, and if so, the illness will be much milder. The chicken-pox vaccine is an example of a live attenuated vaccine, meaning that it contains a weakened form of the varicella–zoster virus it protects against, and live attenuated vaccines are the only type of vaccines that carry this small risk. These are used when studies suggest that the weakened virus packs a far more effective immune punch against infections. Live attenuated vaccines could cause a mild form of infection in extremely rare cases in some children with impaired immunity or HIV, which is why live attenuated vaccines may not be recommended for these children. Some of our own parents intentionally infected us with chicken pox by encouraging us to play with our rashy, feverish siblings or friends. Before the vaccine became widely available in the US in 1995, taking kids to a so-called pox party to catch this illness made sense because children tend to have mild disease and develop immunity to subsequent chicken-pox infections, while adults contracting it for the first time are at higher risk for complications. In other words, the benefits of pox parties seemed to outweigh the long-term risks of catching chicken pox at an older age. Still, chicken pox did come with risks for those of us born before routine vaccination against it. During the first 25 years of the US chicken-pox vaccination program, the vaccine has prevented an estimated 91 million cases, 238,000 hospitalizations, and 2,000 deaths.

Both of my kids have received the chicken-pox vaccine. They didn't get the childhood experience of attending an infectious party like my friends and I did, but they did get a treat postjab.

Another widespread worry surrounds thimerosal, a preservative used in some vaccines. Mercury is a naturally occurring element found in the Earth's crust, air, soil, and water and comes in a few forms. Thimerosal contains ethylmercury, which prevents the growth of harmful pathogens in multidose vials. Methylmercury is the type of mercury found in the environment, including in fish or shellfish. At high exposure levels methylmercury—not ethylmercury—is toxic to people.

Yet another common question is *Why should kids receive the HPV (or human papillomavirus)or hepatitis B vaccines if they're not going to engage in behaviors that put them at increased risk?* Many parents believe that their children don't need these shots.

Public-health agencies around the world agree that hepatitis B vaccination is important. Hepatitis B is a serious liver infection caused by the hep B virus (HBV), which causes 30 million new infections and kills nearly a million annually around the world. Chronic HBV infection can lead to liver cancer and liver cirrhosis and failure. According to the CDC, most children and many adults show no symptoms of the virus but can still spread it to others. Contrary to common belief, HBV is not solely transmitted through sexual contact or drug use. It can also be transmitted by sharing personal items like razors or toothbrushes and may live on objects for seven days or more. The hep B vaccine does not contain any live viruses, which means it can't cause hepatitis B. Extremely rarely, the vaccine may cause allergic reactions. The CDC recommends against vaccinating individuals with a yeast allergy because the proteins used in the vaccine are produced in yeast cells. The most common side effect of the hep B vaccine is a sore arm at the site of injection that lasts for one to two days.

Public-health agencies also agree that the vaccine against HPV is an important way to prevent many cases of cancer. HPV is the most common sexually transmitted disease. According to Planned Parenthood, sexual skin-to-skin contact is all that is required for the transmission of the virus, meaning that a condom will not prevent the transmission of the virus (but it does reduce its transmission). As such, cases of HPV have been observed in people who have not experienced penetrative sexual intercourse. There is also some evidence that the virus can be transmitted at the time of birth. It can't be contracted without skin contact, meaning you can't get it from a hard surface like a doorknob or toilet seat. HPV has been associated with various forms of cancer, including cancers of the cervix, vagina, vulva, penis, anus, rectum, and throat. It's thought that the infection causes about 37,000 cases of cancer per year in the United States.

Talk to your doctor to find out if your children qualify for the vaccine. In general, the CDC recommends that all girls and boys who are eleven or twelve (note that vaccinations can start at nine years of age) receive a series of HPV vaccine. Older unvaccinated individuals may also be eligible. It is best for the vaccine to be given before individuals are exposed to HPV. It is ideal not to wait until becoming sexually active to get vaccinated.

The HPV vaccine does not contain live virus. Some forms of it are contraindicated for people with yeast allergies. Redness and swelling at the injection site are the most common side effects, with rare fainting and temporary movements resembling a seizure, which is why doctors may recommend that people who receive the vaccine lie down for fifteen minutes.

So yeah, all vaccines are different, they reduce risk, and

they're imperfect, but they're a layer of protection that we can give our children. I think of it this way: in a world where our children are constantly exposed to hazards, we can protect them from the worst outcomes of several of those hazards and counting—infectious diseases—with a series of jabs. This kind of honesty seems crucial to changing minds.

You might not need to persuade someone that they should get a vaccine for their kid. You might have more of an impact by lifting a piece of someone's burden. Can you give them a ride, watch their younger child, or go with them to help wrangle a toddler?

Finally, don't expect to change someone's mind about vaccines in one conversation, and know when to stop. People tend to need time to process. Share with a fellow parent why you chose to vaccinate your children. You can share your story with Voices for Vaccines, or direct people with doubts to https://www.voicesfor-vaccines.org/why-i-vax/

And share with parents credible resources to answer their questions, including the CDC at https://www.cdc.gov/vaccines/schedules/ and the AAP at https://www.healthychildren.org/English/safety-prevention/immunizations/

9

doing the right thing

It's my thirteenth year as a co-parent. Life has treated my family well. My children are brilliant and healthy, spending the summer of 2023 with all four of their grandparents, *chithis*, uncles, aunties, cousins, and friends. I still peek at them while they sleep at night, not with extreme anxiety like I did when my first baby was tiny but to relish the moment, with the certainty that this, too, shall pass. I gaze at their sweet faces, feeling joy, appreciation, and exhaustion. My heart is still perpetually anxious with worry about my children and all children. But the anxiety has taken a different form. When my babies were born, I needed to know that their father and I were doing everything we could possibly do to make sure they would always be okay and that they would always live their best lives. It was an overwhelming responsibility that loomed vaguely beyond the horizon. But the time vanished, leaving me repeating the old clichés of count-less generations of parents: *They grow up too fast. In the blink of an eye*. It happens to all of us. I can conjure moments in that span of time, as fleeting as rainbows, in my mind, like singing "You Are My Sunshine" and watching Stompy the Bear night after night, pushing swings day after day, and all of the school drop-offs, kissing them on the cheek and telling them I love them more than anything, willing them to get through the day and come back home.

Having spent the better part of a decade as a science writer covering children and health, I realize that, in many ways, doing everything we can do as parents can be boiled down into a short list: get the best prenatal care possible; get the best health care, including mental health care, possible for children; learn first aid and CPR; make sure to install and use car seats correctly; strap furniture and televisions securely to the walls; beware of batteries and small magnets, unstrapped furniture and outdated window-blind cords wherever you take your small children; feed babies sufficiently and safely; cut grapes into quarters and take other safety precautions around choking hazards; feed kids plenty of fruits and vegetables; avoid pollution; let children be who they are; surround them with trees, beauty, and safe spaces; protect them from bigotry and cops; teach them well. Some of these are so much easier said than done that it's almost funny.

By and large, the most important action, in addition to har-nessing science and social justice to guide our own families, is to keep pushing the people in power to put their weight be-hind making institutions and systems do the right thing. This means not just going through performative motions. There are progressive parents in positions of power everywhere. Always hold yourself and each other accountable. Acting with integrity and in line with the values they purport to hold dear, especially when those actions or inactions affect other human beings, is what people with power need to lose sleep over.

My unearned privileges are immense, and, like anyone else, no matter how hard I try, I will never be able to fathom another person's vast experience and unique perspective. Still, I deeply believe that it's always worth trying. For now, there are a few things I know. You have to love yourself. But you don't have to approve of the views you once held or your past actions. Growth is the opposite of hypocrisy, and remorse is not a bad thing.

Punch up. Secure your own well-being and your children's first, but once that's ensured as much as possible, expend available bandwidth on all kids. Use any leverage you have, including your community's resources, to hold the system accountable for everyone's health.

For some progressive parents, one elephant in the room is religion. Some progressives believe that religion is the singular enemy, the fundamental reason for racism, misogyny, the patriarchy, and the continued erosion of our rights. There's no doubt that religious justification for widespread oppression and nationalism has been a major source of real harm to children and families in the United States and worldwide. Religion has been used to justify mass enslavement and genocide based on hierarchy and hate. Groups who fight for justice via the fight for the separation of church and state are fighting a crucial fight.

At the same time, I'm convinced that religion is not the singular enemy. Eliminating religion will not eliminate everything that oppresses our children. I know many religious and non-religious parents who share a deep belief in equity, justice, and science. I also know many deeply bigoted, science-denying religious folks and many deeply bigoted, science-denying atheists. There are sects of nearly all religious and nonreligious groups that seek to exclude or oppress women and girls, LGBTQ+ folks, people of certain races and ethnicities, people with disabilities, and other groups of historically-marginalized people.

Keira Havens, the scientist who often warns of the harms of biological essentialism, says that religion can seem like "the easy button to hierarchy" because of the idea behind "God's plan in nature." But "removing religion is no guarantee" that humans will "start to think of ourselves as true equals," she tells me.

We've "already shaped our society to reflect hierarchical power dynamics and those patterns," and those "systems will perpetuate unless we actively dismantle them."

Dehumanization, biological essentialism, and hate are the root of evil. Over the past decade, I've realized that, throughout history, science (and how its findings are translated into policy and practice) is sometimes as dramatic and hilarious as it is dark, infuriating, and heartbreaking. There are rifts, power grabs, egos, and epic showdowns that can span generations. And there have always been parents on all sides.

Life is rough for a lot of families. The future seems pretty bleak. In the United States, since surpassing deaths from automobile accidents in 2020, guns have become the leading cause of death in children and teens (as SciParent Layla Katiraee says, there's "no sugarcoating" that owning a gun increases the risk of children being injured or killed, even when the gun is stored safely). Despair is widespread, and it's no surprise that this bleakness is hurting children. More and more children are dying by suicide. The disconnect between the messaging that suggests that it's important for children to seek mental-health support and the dire lack of mental-health professionals, psychotherapists, and psychiatrists is mind-boggling. My daughter laments to me that all too often, children are told to "go for a walk" or "meditate" to deal with their mental health. Walks and mediation can be lovely, but they're no stand-in for evidence-based support from trained professionals.

As a mentally ill science journalist who has covered mental illness extensively, another thing I know and cannot repeat enough is that mentally ill people are absolutely not the cause of gun violence and mass shootings. This fallacious belief, uncritically repeated across the media, harms children and families. Mentally ill people are far more likely to be harmed by stigma and guns than to commit gun violence, and that's a fact. The American Academy of Pediatrics provides a one-stop resource to increase safety and reduce risk in the home and out at play, including gun safety, choking hazards, and more, at https://www. healthychildren.org/English/safety-prevention.

Another thing that matters is parents breaking up their cliques and expanding their circles to build community. New research on friendship and economic mobility suggests that people are most likely to be friends with people of a similar socioeconomic status, especially at the top of the ladder. Economic connectedness, which is a measure of the extent of friendships across class lines, boosts social mobility and the well-being of all people, including children.

All of the social and scientific constructs that seek to slot humans into biological categories, from genitals to sex chromosomes to race, are based on how the observers in power see the world. Science has traditionally sought to partition life. Modern science has only now begun to accept that, in reality, hierarchies and categories are more of a reflection of our instinct to categorize than reality.

In addition to ableist words, there are also ableist ideals. For instance, consider the very idea of productivity, concerted ambition, and hard work as universal ideals, all in the pursuit of specific measures of success. In America, we're indoctrinated with the notion that setting specific goals—around education, career, income, weight, relationships, accolades, and more—and working hard to achieve them is the one virtuous life path. The adults dish out different versions of the same question to children: *What do you want to be when you grow up?* The answer to that question can seem essential. Scratch the surface, and this seemingly benign and ostensibly laudable notion is a ploy of capitalism and the police state. That might sound extreme, but at best, it leaves little room for children to explore the world, learn who they are, develop their values, and simply be. The ideal of individual ambition and hard work as the path to financial security, well-being, comfort, and happiness justifies oppression. It relies unrealistically on the myth of a path of universal upward mobility, weighing disproportionately on the most marginalized, as if the resilience of generations that have survived oppression and genocide is a hallmark of character rather than a means of survival. It tacitly reinforces the violent idea that those who are housing- or food-insecure deserve their lot in life. It erases the truth that productivity is not the same as the pursuit of happiness.

None of this is to say children shouldn't set goals for themselves and strive to reach them. We all should. There's perhaps no better feeling than seeing a child take pride in an accomplishment. As author and lawyer Meena Harris (niece of Vice President Kamala Harris) suggests in a 2023 essay for *Parents*, kids can be ambitious without having to "pick a career." None of this is to say that adulthood isn't coming for all of our children, and they need to be prepared. But I've come to worry less about achievement and more about examining our relationship to ambition and rugged individualism as parents.

No, we're not a monolith, but what can progressive parents do that ties our values of science and justice together? Know that we've always been one humanity. Not that long ago, those who weren't free to be their most expansive selves surely thought of future generations and wondered whether we would be free. Raising our children to be their most authentic, expansive selves is a testament to that human penchant to have hope and love for the children who will take the mantle, in our own lifetimes, and generations after our bodies have returned to dust and our spirits released into the universe.

★ ★ ★ ★ ★

Acknowledgments

I couldn't have written this book without my spouse Jesse encouraging me, holding down the fort, and feeding my face, among the countless other ways you offered support. Thank you for always helping me collect the candy I need to evolve.

I'm eternally grateful to my kids' amichi and ayya (Roopa and Periannan Senapathy), and nana and grandpa (Laurie Baruch and Joe Milinovich), the best grandparents on Earth. This book wouldn't have happened without you. It's a gift to watch our babies grow up with you by their side.

A special thanks to the dear friends who keep me grounded, and who hold space with me when reality becomes overwhelming.

To Matte Black for all of the early reading, and the necessary validation and VCs alike.

This book is the aerial view of all of the patterns and stories I've gleaned since I first started blogging in 2012. I appreciate my editors and production team at Hanover Square for believing in the vision and cheering it on to the finish line.

I owe the universe for bringing Chris Bucci into my DMs. Thanks, Chris, for seeing the value in my ideas and empowering me to pursue them. Megan Thee Stallion herself would be lucky to have an agent like you.

To my fellow Grounded Parents and Skepchicks and our unbreakable spirit of curiosity.

To the folks at SciShow for the opportunity to work on such accessible, fascinating, rigorous, digestible, and fun content with awesome editors and team members. Working with you all is always a privilege and a legitimately enjoyable learning experience.

To the wise teachers, editors, writers, and various other badasses who have generously advised me over the years.

To the organizations that provide resources to advance the work of science writers and journalists.

To the ones who tried to erase me, thank you for making me stronger.

To those who fight for our children.

To our trillion ancestors and their future descendants, with love.

References

1: the progressive parent's dilemma

Pelham, Victoria. "The Difference between Postpartum Anxiety, OCD and Psychosis." *Cedars-Sinai Blog*, May 2, 2023. https://www.cedars-sinai. org/blog/difference-between-postpartum-anxiety-ocd-psychosis.html.

US Politics & Policy. "Beyond Red vs. Blue: The Political Typology." *Pew Research Center*. November 9, 2021. https://www.pewresearch.org/topic/ politics-policy/political-parties-polarization/political-typology/.

Taylor, Chris. "How One Woman's Yard Sign Became a Rallying Cry for Allies." *Mashable*, June 16, 2020. https://mashable.com/article/in-this-house- we-believe-black-lives-matter-kindness-is-everything-sign.

hooks, bell. *Ain't I a Woman: Black Women and Feminism*. Boston, MA: South End Press, 1981.

Crenshaw, Kimberlé W. *On Intersectionality: Essential Writings*. New York, NY: The New Press, 2017.

Online Public Health. "Equity vs. Equality: What's the Difference?" November 5, 2020. *George Washington University*. Accessed September 13, 2023. https://onlinepublichealth.gwu.edu/resources/equity-vs-equality/.

"0002, Brutal and Relentless." *Dinosaur Couch*, 2022. https://twitter.com/dinosaurcouch/status/1540052892362702850.

Claremon, Mirei Takashima. "The Cognitive Bias That Prevents America from Addressing Mass Shootings." *An Injustice!*, July 4, 2022. https://aninjusticemag.com/the-cognitive-bias-that-prevents-america-from-addressing-mass-shootings-c29a29089e98.

Dean, Kristy K., and Anne M. Koenig. "Cross-Cultural Differences and Similarities in Attribution." Edited by Kenneth Keith. *Cross-Cultural Psychology: Contemporary Themes and Perspectives*, Second Edition. March 25, 2019, 575–97. https://doi.org/10.1002/9781119519348.ch28.

Sullivan, Dylan, and Jason Hickel. "Capitalism and Extreme Poverty: A Global Analysis of Real Wages, Human Height, and Mortality since the Long 16th Century." *World Development* 161 (January 1, 2023): 106026. https://doi.org/10.1016/j.worlddev.2022.106026.

Hickel, Jason. "Bill Gates Says Poverty Is Decreasing. He Couldn't Be More Wrong." *The Guardian*, January 29, 2019. https://www.theguardian.com/commentisfree/2019/jan/29/bill-gates-davos-global-poverty-infographic-neoliberal.

Roser, Max. "The Short History of Global Living Conditions and Why It Matters That We Know It." *Our World in Data*. Accessed September 14, 2023. https://ourworldindata.org/a-history-of-global-living-conditions.

"Ho-Chunk Nation." *Wisconsin First Nations*. Accessed September 14, 2023. https://wisconsinfirstnations.org/ho-chunk-nation/.

Sears, William, Martha Sears, Robert Sears, and James Sears. *The Baby Book, Revised Edition: Everything You Need to Know about Your Baby from Birth to Age Two*. Little, Brown Spark, 2013.

2: healthy scrutiny of science

Leshner, Alan. "Trust in Science Is Not the Problem." *Issues in Science and Technology*, May 2021. https://issues.org/trust-in-science-is-not-the-problem-engagement-leshner/.

Lopez-Carmen, Victor A., Janya McCalman, Tessa Benveniste, Deborah Askew, Geoffrey Spurling, Erika Langham, and Roxanne Bainbridge. "Working Together to Improve the Mental Health of Indigenous Children: A Systematic Review." *Children and Youth Services Review* 104 (September 2019): 104408. https://doi.org/10.1016/j.childyouth.2019.104408.

Kahan, Dan M., Asheley R. Landrum, Katie Carpenter, Laura Helft, and Kathleen Hall Jamieson. "Science Curiosity and Political Information Processing." *Political Psychology* 38 (January 26, 2017): 179–99. https://doi.org/10.1111/pops.12396.

Motta, Matthew, Daniel Chapman, Kathryn Haglin, and Dan M. Kahan. "Reducing the Administrative Demands of the Science Curiosity Scale: A Validation Study." *International Journal of Public Opinion Research* 33, no. 2 (December 2019): 215–33. https://doi.org/10.1093/ijpor/edz049.

"Key Findings about Americans' Confidence in Science and Their Views of Scientists' Role in Society." *Pew Research Center.* February 12, 2020. https://www.pewresearch.org/short-reads/2020/02/12/key-findings-about-americans-confidence-in-science-and-their-views-on-scientists-role-in-society/.

Hepburn, Brian and Hanne Andersen, "Scientific Method," *The Stanford Encyclopedia of Philosophy* (Summer 2021 Edition), Edward N. Zalta (ed.). https://plato.stanford.edu/archives/sum2021/entries/scientific-method/.

UC Museum of Paleontology Understanding Science. "Understanding Science." Understanding Science - How Science REALLY Works. Accessed October 22, 2023. https://undsci.berkeley.edu/.

The Australian National University. "Incorporating Indigenous Knowledge into Your Teaching." *Living Knowledge*, 2008. Accessed September 14, 2023. https://livingknowledge.anu.edu.au/html/educators/02_questions.htm.

Sidik, Saima. "Weaving Indigenous Knowledge into the Scientific Method." *Nature* 601, no. 7892 (January 2022): 285–87. https://doi.org/10.1038/d41586-022-00029-2.

Evenhouse, Eirik, and Siobhan Reilly. "Improved Estimates of the Benefits of Breastfeeding Using Sibling Comparisons to Reduce Selection Bias." Health Services Research, December 1, 2005. https://doi.org/10.1111/j.1475-6773.2004.00453.x.

Binns, Colin, MiKyung Lee, and Wah Yun Low. "The Long-Term Public Health Benefits of Breastfeeding." *Asia Pacific Journal of Public Health* 28, no. 1 (January 1, 2016): 7–14. https://doi.org/10.1177/1010539515624964.

Pérez-Escamilla, Rafael, Josefa L. Martinez, and Sofia Segura-Pérez. "Impact of the Baby-Friendly Hospital Initiative on Breastfeeding and Child Health Outcomes: A Systematic Review." *Maternal and Child Nutrition* 12, no. 3 (2016): 402–17. https://doi.org/10.1111/mcn.12294.

Senapathy, Kavin. "Is Breastfeeding Really Best and Is Formula Harmful?" *SciMoms*, February 4, 2019.

Leung, Alexander K. C., and Reginald S. Sauve. "Breast Is Best for Babies." *Journal of the National Medical Association* 97, no. 7 (July 2005): 1010–1019. https://www.ncbi.nlm.nih.gov/pmc/articles/PMC2569316/.

Meek, Joan Younger, and Lawrence Noble. "Policy Statement: Breastfeeding and the Use of Human Milk." *Pediatrics* 150, no. 1 (June 27, 2022). https://doi.org/10.1542/peds.2022-057988.

Black, Robert E., Harold Alderman, Zulfiqar Ahmed Bhutta, Stuart Gillespie, Lawrence Haddad, Susan Horton, Anna Lartey, et al. "Maternal and Child Nutrition: Building Momentum for Impact." *The Lancet* 382, no. 9890 (August 3, 2013): 372–75. https://doi.org/10.1016/s0140-6736(13)60988-5.

Hewlett, Barry S., and Steve Winn. "Allomaternal Nursing in Humans." *Current Anthropology* 55, no. 2 (April 1, 2014): 200–229. https://doi.org/10.1086/675657.

Stevens, Emily E., Thelma E. Patrick, and Rita H. Pickler. "A History of Infant Feeding." *Journal of Perinatal Education* 18, no. 2 (January 1, 2009): 32–39. https://doi.org/10.1624/105812409x426314.

Dailey, Kate. "Breastfeeding: Was There Ever a Golden Age?" *BBC News*, January 7, 2014. https://www.bbc.com/news/magazine-25629934.

Cevasco, Carla. "What Parents Did before Baby Formula." *The Atlantic*, May 18, 2022. https://www.theatlantic.com/ideas/archive/2022/05/baby-formula-breastfeeding-history/629889/.

Gannon, Megan. "What Was in Prehistoric Baby Bottles? Now We Know." *National Geographic*, September 2019. https://www.nationalgeographic.com/culture/article/what-in-prehistoric-baby-bottles-now-know-animal-milk.

Vilar-Compte, Mireya, and Rafael Pérez-Escamilla. "Interventions and Policy Approaches to Promote Equity in Breastfeeding." *International Journal for Equity in Health* 21, no. 63 (May 10, 2022). https://doi.org/10.1186/s12939-022-01670-z.

"How Milk Gets from Breast to Baby." In *Baby-Friendly Hospital Initiative: Revised, Updated and Expanded for Integrated Care*. Geneva: World Health Organization, 2009. https://www.ncbi.nlm.nih.gov/books/NBK153490/.

Muller, Mike. "The Baby Killer: A War on Want Investigation into the

Promotion and Sale of Powdered Baby Milks in the Third World." London: *War on Want*, March 1974. https://waronwant.org/resources/baby-killer.

Solomon, Stephen. "The Controversy over Infant Formula." *The New York Times Magazine*, December 6, 1981. Accessed October 12, 2023. https://www.nytimes.com/1981/12/06/magazine/the-controversy-over-infant-formula.html.

"International Code of Marketing of Breast-Milk Substitutes." *World Health Organization*. January 27, 1981. https://www.who.int/publications/i/item/9241541601.

"10 Steps & International Code: The Ten Steps to Successful Breastfeeding." *Baby-Friendly USA*. Accessed September 15, 2023. https://www.baby-friendlyusa.org/for-facilities/practice-guidelines/10-steps-and-international-code/.

USFDA. "FDA Evaluation of Infant Formula Response." *US Food And Drug Administration*, September 2022. https://www.fda.gov/media/161689/download.

Weston, Jennifer. "Water Is Life: The Rise of the Mní Wičóni Movement." Cultural Survival, 2017. Accessed September 19, 2023. https://www.culturalsurvival.org/publications/cultural-survival-quarterly/water-life-rise-mni-wiconi-movement.

Gregory, Katherine, and W. Allan Walker. "Immunologic Factors in Human Milk and Disease Prevention in the Preterm Infant." *Current Pediatrics Reports* 1, (September 26, 2013): 222–28. https://doi.org/10.1007/s40124-013-0028-2.

Hariton, Eduardo, and Joseph J. Locascio. "Randomised Controlled Trials: The Gold Standard for Effectiveness Research." *BJOG: An International Journal of Obstetrics and Gynaecology* 125, no. 13 (December 2018): 1716. https://doi.org/10.1111/1471-0528.15199.

Madigan Library. "Research Guides: Evidence-Based Medicine: Observational Studies." *Penn College of Technology*. Accessed September 15, 2023. https://pct.libguides.com/ebm/clinical-research/observational-studies.

Tulchinsky, Theodore H., and Elena A. Varavikova. "Chapter 3: Measuring, Monitoring, and Evaluating the Health of a Population." In *The New Public Health*, Third Edition, 91–147. Academic Press, 2014. https://doi.org/10.1016/b978-0-12-415766-8.00003-3.

Institute of Medicine (US) Committee on the Evaluation of the Addition of Ingredients New to Infant Formula. "Comparing Infant Formulas with Human Milk." In *Infant Formula: Evaluating the Safety of New Ingredients*, Third Edition. National Academies Press (US), 2004. https://www.ncbi.nlm.nih.gov/books/NBK215837/.

Boone, Kelly M., Jaclyn M. Dynia, Jessica Logan, and Kelly M. Purtell. "Socioeconomic Determinants of Breastfeeding Initiation and Continuation for Families Living in Poverty." *Pediatrics* 144, no. 2_MeetingAbstract (2019): 272. https://doi.org/10.1542/peds.144.2ma3.272.

Orosz, Brooke. "The Lancet: Nonexistent Magic Breasts Could Save 800,000 Lives per Year." *Fed Is Best Foundation*, July 5, 2017. https://fedisbest.org/2017/07/the-lancet-nonexistent-magic-breasts-could-save-800000-lives-per-year/.

Colen, Cynthia G., and David M. Ramey. "Is Breast Truly Best? Estimating the Effects of Breastfeeding on Long-Term Child Health and Wellbeing in the United States Using Sibling Comparisons." *Social Science & Medicine* 109 (May 1, 2014): 55–65. https://doi.org/10.1016/j.socscimed.2014.01.027.

Kramer, Michael S., Beverley Chalmers, Ellen Hodnett, Zinaida Sevkovskaya, Irina Dzikovich, Stanley H. Shapiro, Jean-Paul Collet, et al. "Promotion of Breastfeeding Intervention Trial (PROBIT): A Randomized Trial in the Republic of Belarus." *JAMA* 285, no. 4 (January 24, 2001): 413–20. https://doi.org/10.1001/jama.285.4.413.

Yang, Seungmi, Richard M. Martin, Emily Oken, Mikhail Hameza, Glen M. Doniger, Shimon Amit, Rita Patel, et al. "Breastfeeding during Infancy and Neurocognitive Function in Adolescence: 16-Year Follow-up of the PROBIT Cluster-Randomized Trial." *PLOS Medicine* 15, no. 4 (April 20, 2018): e1002554. https://doi.org/10.1371/journal.pmed.1002554.

Dewey, Kathryn G., Laurie A. Nommsen-Rivers, M. Jane Heinig, and Roberta J. Cohen. "Risk Factors for Suboptimal Infant Breastfeeding Behavior, Delayed Onset of Lactation, and Excess Neonatal Weight Loss." *Pediatrics* 112, no. 3 (September 1, 2003): 607–19. https://doi.org/10.1542/peds.112.3.607.

Del Castillo-Hegyi, Christie, Jennifer Achilles, B. Jody Segrave-Daly, and Lynnette Hafken. "Fatal Hypernatremic Dehydration in a Term Exclusively Breastfed Newborn." *Children* 9, no. 9 (September 13, 2022): 1379. https://doi.org/10.3390/children9091379.

Miyoshi, Yasuhiro, Hideyo Suenaga, Mikihiro Aoki, and Shigeki Tanaka. "Determinants of Excessive Weight Loss in Breastfed Full-Term Newborns at a Baby-Friendly Hospital: A Retrospective Cohort Study." *International Breastfeeding Journal* 15, no. 19 (March 24, 2020). https://doi.org/10.1186/s13006-020-00263-2.

Whitten, Allison. "Do IQ Tests Actually Measure Intelligence?" *Discover Magazine*, July 1, 2020. https://www.discovermagazine.com/mind/do-iq-tests-actually-measure-intelligence.

Duckworth, Angela, Patrick D. Quinn, Donald R. Lynam, Rolf Loeber, and Magda Stouthamer-Loeber. "Role of Test Motivation in Intelligence Testing." *Proceedings of the National Academy of Sciences of the United States of America*, 108, no. 19 (April 25, 2011): 7716–20. https://doi.org/10.1073/pnas.1018601108.

Ghosh, Ranjini. "Safe Infant Feeding: Parents Aren't Getting the Information They Need." *SciMoms*, August 6, 2020.

Segrave-Daly, Jody. "How to Breastfeed during the First 2 Weeks of Life." *The New York Times*, April 18, 2020. https://www.nytimes.com/article/breastfeeding-newborn.html.

CDC. "How to Keep Your Breast Pump Clean." In Water, Sanitation, and Environmentally Related Hygiene. *Centers for Disease Control and Prevention*. Accessed September 15, 2023. https://www.cdc.gov/hygiene/childcare/breast-pump.html.

CDC. "How to Prepare and Store Powdered Infant Formula." *Centers for Disease Control and Prevention*. Accessed September 15, 2023. https://www.cdc.gov/nutrition/downloads/prepare-store-powered-infant-formula-508.pdf.

3: revealing the gender and sex lie

Brogan, Dylan. "Vicki McKenna Promotes False Claim about 'Furries' in Waunakee School District." *Isthmus Madison, Wisconsin*, April 4, 2022. https://isthmus.com/news/news/vicki-mckenna-promotes-false-claim/.

Lia Russell, Bangor Daily News. "No, Maine Students Aren't Using Litter Boxes in School." *WGME*, May 20, 2022. https://wgme.com/news/local/no-maine-students-arent-using-litter-boxes-in-school-misinformation-brewer-school-department-tiktok-false-allegations-furries.

Taylor, Kandiss. "The furry days are over when I'm governor…" *Twitter*, March 3, 2022. https://twitter.com/KandissTaylor/status/1506603753008472064.

Evon, Dan. "'Furry Protocol'? False Rumors Circulate about Wisconsin Schools." *Snopes*, April 5, 2022. https://www.snopes.com/fact-check/furry-protocol-wisconsin/.

"Guidance & Policies to Support Transgender, Non-Binary & Gender Expansive Students." *Madison Metropolitan School District*, April 2018. https://resources.finalsite.net/images/v1625663725/madisonk12wius/m5x-6tox6rhrufthykn30/guidancebooklet.pdf.

Zoledziowski, Anya. "The Future of Trans Rights Is on the Ballot." *Vice*, November 7, 2022. https://www.vice.com/en/article/qjkn5q/trans-rights-midterms-2022.

"All Black Lives Matter: Mental Health of Black LGBTQ Youth." *The Trevor Project*. October 6, 2020. https://www.thetrevorproject.org/research-briefs/all-black-lives-matter-mental-health-of-black-lgbtq-youth/.

"Understanding Gender." *Gender Spectrum*. Accessed September 15, 2023. https://www.genderspectrum.org/resources.

PolitiFact. "Why It's Not 'Grooming': What Research Says about Gender and Sexuality in Schools." May 11, 2022. Accessed September 15, 2023. https://www.politifact.com/article/2022/may/11/why-its-not-grooming-what-research-says-about-gend/.

"The Misia Pledge," 2020. *Diversity Pride*. Accessed September 15, 2023. https://diversitypride.org/misiapledge.html.

"What's Transphobia, Also Called Transmisia?" *Planned Parenthood*. Accessed September 15, 2023. https://www.plannedparenthood.org/learn/gender-identity/transgender/whats-transphobia.

GSA Network. "Beyond the Binary: A Tool Kit for Gender Identity Activism in Schools." *GSA Network, Transgender Law Center*, and *National Center for Lesbian Rights*. Accessed September 15, 2023. https://gsanetwork.org/wp-content/uploads/2019/04/BeyondtheBinary-v2.pdf.

Montañez, Amanda. "Visualizing Sex as a Spectrum." *Scientific American Blog Network*, August 29, 2017. https://blogs.scientificamerican.com/sa-visual/visualizing-sex-as-a-spectrum/.

Human Rights Campaign. "Glossary of Terms." *HRC Foundation*. Accessed September 15, 2023. https://www.hrc.org/resources/glossary-of-terms.

"LGBTQ+ Glossary." *It Gets Better Project.* Accessed September 15, 2023. https://itgetsbetter.org/glossary/.

Mills, Emily. "Madison Prepares to Counter-Program the TERFs." *Tone Madison*, March 29, 2022. https://tonemadison.com/articles/madison-prepares-to-counter-program-the-terfs/.

Parker, Kim, Juliana Menasce Horowitz, and Anna Brown. "Americans' Complex Views on Gender Identity and Transgender Issues." *Pew Research Center's Social & Demographic Trends Project.* June 28, 2022. https://www.pewresearch.org/social-trends/2022/06/28/americans-complex-views-on-gender-identity-and-transgender-issues/.

Preves, Sharon. "Negotiating the Constraints of Gender Binarism: Intersexuals' Challenge to Gender Categorization." *Current Sociology* 48, no. 3 (July 1, 2000): 27–50. https://doi.org/10.1177/0011392100048003004.

Havens, Keira. "Box of Rocks #1—Rocks Having Sex." *Medium*, November 22, 2022. Accessed September 15, 2023. https://medium.com/@Keira_Havens/box-of-rocks-b8aec0c8710e.

Laudan, Rachel. *From Mineralogy to Geology: The Foundations of a Science, 1650–1830.* University of Chicago Press, 1987.

DuBois, L. Zachary, and Heather Shattuck-Heidorn. "Challenging the Binary: Gender/Sex and the Bio-logics of Normalcy." *American Journal of Human Biology* 33, no. 5 (June 6, 2021). https://doi.org/10.1002/ajhb.23623.

Karkazis, Katrina. "The Misuses of 'Biological Sex.'" *The Lancet* 394, no. 10212 (November 23, 2019): 1898–99. https://doi.org/10.1016/s0140-6736(19)32764-3.

Ritz, Stacey A., and Lorraine Greaves. "Transcending the Male–Female Binary in Biomedical Research: Constellations, Heterogeneity, and Mechanism When Considering Sex and Gender." *International Journal of Environmental Research and Public Health* 19, no. 7 (March 30, 2022): 4083. https://doi.org/10.3390/ijerph19074083.

Fausto-Sterling, Anne. "The Bare Bones of Sex: Part 1—Sex and Gender." *Signs: Journal of Women in Culture and Society* 30, no. 2 (January 1, 2005): 1491–1527. https://doi.org/10.1086/424932.

Joel, Daphna. "Genetic-Gonadal-Genitals Sex (3G-Sex) and the Misconception of Brain and Gender, or, Why 3G-Males and 3G-Females Have

Intersex Brain and Intersex Gender." *Biology of Sex Differences* 3, no. 1 (January 1, 2012): 27. https://doi.org/10.1186/2042-6410-3-27.

Carey, Sarah B., Laramie Aközbek, and Alex Harkess. "The Contributions of Nettie Stevens to the Field of Sex Chromosome Biology." *Philosophical Transactions of the Royal Society B* 377, no. 1850 (March 21, 2022). https://doi.org/10.1098/rstb.2021.0215.

Miko, Ilona. "Gregor Mendel and the Principles of Inheritance." *Nature Education*, 1, no. 1 (2008): 134. https://www.nature.com/scitable/topicpage/gregor-mendel-and-the-principles-of-inheritance-593/.

Bachtrog, Doris, Judith E. Mank, Catherine L. Peichel, Mark Kirkpatrick, Sarah P. Otto, Tia-Lynn Ashman, Matthew W. Hahn, et al. "Sex Determination: Why So Many Ways of Doing It?" *PLOS Biology* 12, no. 7 (July 1, 2014): e1001899. https://doi.org/10.1371/journal.pbio.1001899.

"Humane Genetics: Towards a More Humane Genetics Education." *BSCS Science Learning.* Accessed September 15, 2023. https://bscs.org/humane-genetics/.

Furman, Benjamin L. S., David C. H. Metzger, Iulia Darolti, Alison E. Wright, Benjamin A. Sandkam, Pedro Almeida, Jacelyn J. Shu, and Judith E. Mank. "Sex Chromosome Evolution: So Many Exceptions to the Rules." *Genome Biology and Evolution* 12, no. 6 (April 21, 2020): 750–63. https://doi.org/10.1093/gbe/evaa081.

Clancy, Suzanne, and William Brown. "Translation: DNA to mRNA to Protein." *Nature Education*, 1, no. 1 (2008): 101. https://www.nature.com/scitable/topicpage/translation-dna-to-mrna-to-protein-393/.

Costello, Cary. "The Phalloclitoris: Anatomy and Ideology." *The Intersex Roadshow* (blog), January 31, 2011. Accessed September 15, 2023. https://intersexroadshow.blogspot.com/2011/01/phalloclitoris-anatomy-and-ideology.html.

Koopman, Peter, John Gubbay, Nigel Vivian, Peter N. Goodfellow, and Robin Lovell-Badge. "Male Development of Chromosomally Female Mice Transgenic for *Sry.*" *Nature* 351, no. 6322 (May 1, 1991): 117–21. https://doi.org/10.1038/351117a0.

interACT. "Intersex Variations Glossary: People-Centered Definitions of Intersex Traits & Variations in Sex Characteristics." *interACT Advocates for Intersex Youth.* Accessed September 19, 2023. https://interactadvocates.org/wp-content/uploads/2022/10/Intersex-Variations-Glossary.pdf.

Ainsworth, Claire. "Sex Redefined." *Nature* 518, no. 7539 (February 1, 2015): 288–91. https://doi.org/10.1038/518288a.

Eliot, Lise, Adnan Ahmed, Hiba Khan, and Julie Patel. "Dump the 'Dimorphism': Comprehensive Synthesis of Human Brain Studies Reveals Few Male-Female Differences beyond Size." *Neuroscience & Biobehavioral Reviews* 125 (June 1, 2021): 667–97. https://doi.org/10.1016/j.neubiorev.2021.02.026.

Adjepong, Anima, and Travers. "The Problem with Sex Segregated Sport." *The Society Pages: Engaging Sports*. December 9, 2022. https://thesocietypages.org/engagingsports/2022/12/09/the-problem-with-sex-segregated-sport/.

Mertens, Maggie. "Separating Sports by Sex Doesn't Make Sense: The Case for Coed Sports." *The Atlantic*, September 17, 2022. https://www.theatlantic.com/culture/archive/2022/09/sports-gender-sex-segregation-coed/671460/.

Rioux, Charlie, Scott Weedon, Kira London-Nadeau, Ash Paré, Robert-Paul Juster, Leslie E. Roos, Makayla Freeman, and Lianne Tomfohr-Madsen. "Gender-Inclusive Writing for Epidemiological Research on Pregnancy." *Journal of Epidemiology and Community Health* 76, no. 9 (June 28, 2022): 823–27. https://doi.org/10.1136/jech-2022-219172.

Brown, Anna. "About 5% of Young Adults in the US Say Their Gender Is Different from Their Sex Assigned at Birth." *Pew Research Center*. June 7, 2022. https://www.pewresearch.org/short-reads/2022/06/07/about-5-of-young-adults-in-the-u-s-say-their-gender-is-different-from-their-sex-assigned-at-birth/.

Ashley, Florence. "A Critical Commentary on 'Rapid-Onset Gender Dysphoria.'" *The Sociological Review* 68, no. 4 (July 1, 2020): 779–99. https://doi.org/10.1177/0038026120934693.

Bauer, Greta R., Margaret L. Lawson, and Daniel L. Metzger. "Do Clinical Data from Transgender Adolescents Support the Phenomenon of 'Rapid Onset Gender Dysphoria'?" *The Journal of Pediatrics* 243 (November 15, 2021: 224-227.e2. https://doi.org/10.1016/j.jpeds.2021.11.020.

"Puberty Blockers for Transgender and Gender-Diverse Youth." *Mayo Clinic*. Accessed September 15, 2023. https://www.mayoclinic.org/diseases-conditions/gender-dysphoria/in-depth/pubertal-blockers/art-20459075.

Human Rights Campaign. "Get the Facts on Gender-Affirming Care." *HRC Foundation*. Accessed September 15, 2023. https://www.hrc.org/resources/get-the-facts-on-gender-affirming-care.

4: beginning to navigate race, ethnicity, and ancestry

Spicuzza, Mary. "What to Know about the Forward Statue That Was Toppled during Madison Protests." *Milwaukee Journal Sentinel*, June 25, 2020. https://www.jsonline.com/story/news/politics/2020/06/24/madison-protests-what-know-forward-statue-toppled/3249239001/.

Bartick, Melissa, Briana J. Jegier, Brittany D. Green, Eleanor Bimla Schwarz, Arnold Reinhold, and Alison M. Stuebe. "Disparities in Breastfeeding: Impact on Maternal and Child Health Outcomes and Costs." *The Journal of Pediatrics* 181 (February 1, 2017): 49–55. e6. https://doi.org/10.1016/j.jpeds.2016.10.028.

Braveman, Paula, Elaine Bratic Arkin, Dwayne Proctor, Tina J. Kauh, and Nicole Holm. "Systemic and Structural Racism: Definitions, Examples, Health Damages, and Approaches to Dismantling." *Health Affairs* 41, no. 2 (February 1, 2022): 171–78. https://doi.org/10.1377/hlthaff.2021.01394.

Mwitynski, Max. "What Is Tree Equity? A New Tool from UChicago Data Scientists Is Helping to Transform Neighborhood Health." *UChicago News*, November 23, 2021. https://news.uchicago.edu/story/what-tree-equity-new-tool-uchicago-data-scientists-helping-transform-neighborhood-health.

Senapathy, Kavin. "The Black Box Breakers." *Grow*, 2021. https://www.grow-byginkgo.com/2021/10/21/the-black-box-breakers/.

Saini, Angela. *Superior : The Return of Race Science*. Beacon Press, 2019. https://www.penguinrandomhouse.com/books/607248/superior-by-angela-saini/.

Hill, Latoya, Samantha Artiga, and Usha Ranji. "Racial Disparities in Maternal and Infant Health: Current Status and Efforts to Address Them." *KFF*. November 1, 2022. https://www.kff.org/racial-equity-and-health-policy/issue-brief/racial-disparities-in-maternal-and-infant-health-current-status-and-efforts-to-address-them/.

Alson, Julianna G., Whitney R. Robinson, LaShawnDa Pittman, and Kemi M. Doll. "Incorporating Measures of Structural Racism into Population Studies of Reproductive Health in the United States: A Narrative Review." *Health Equity* 5, no. 1 (February 25, 2021): 49–58. https://doi.org/10.1089/heq.2020.0081.

Boyd, Rhea, Edwin Lindo, Lachelle Weeks, and Monica McLemore. "On Racism: A New Standard for Publishing on Racial Health Inequities." *Health Affairs*, July 2, 2020. https://doi.org/10.1377/forefront.20200630.939347.

Hardeman, Rachel R., Eduardo Medina, and Katy B. Kozhimannil. "Structural Racism and Supporting Black Lives—The Role of Health Professionals." *The New England Journal of Medicine* 375, no. 22 (December 1, 2016): 2113–15. https://doi.org/10.1056/nejmp1609535.

Miller, Claire Cain, Sarah Kliff, and Larry Buchanan. "Childbirth Is Deadlier for Black Families Even When They're Rich, Expansive Study Finds." *The New York Times*, February 12, 2023. https://www.nytimes.com/interactive/2023/02/12/upshot/child-maternal-mortality-rich-poor.html.

Williams, Melissa J., and Jennifer L. Eberhardt. "Biological Conceptions of Race and the Motivation to Cross Racial Boundaries." *Journal of Personality and Social Psychology* 94, no. 6 (January 1, 2008): 1033–47. https://doi.org/10.1037/0022-3514.94.6.1033.

Tsai, Jennifer J. "How Should Educators and Publishers Eliminate Racial Essentialism?" *AMA Journal of Ethics* 24, no. 3 (March 1, 2022): E201–11. https://doi.org/10.1001/amajethics.2022.201.

Larrimore, Mark. "Antinomies of Race: Diversity and Destiny in Kant." *Patterns of Prejudice* 42, no. 4-5 (2008): 341–63. doi:10.1080/00313220802377313.

Kendi, Ibram X. *How to Be an Antiracist*. One World, 2019.

Center on the Developing Child. "How Racism Can Affect Child Development." *Harvard University*. Accessed September 15, 2023. https://developingchild.harvard.edu/resources/racism-and-ecd/.

Jorde, Lynn B., and Stephen Wooding. "Genetic Variation, Classification and 'Race.'" *Nature Genetics* 36, Suppl. 11 (October 26, 2004): S28–33. https://doi.org/10.1038/ng1435.

Hiernaux, Jean, and Michael Banton. *Four Statements on the Race Question*. UNESCO, 1969. https://unesdoc.unesco.org/ark:/48223/pf0000122962.

Trent, Maria, Danielle G. Dooley, and Jacqueline Dougé. "The Impact of Racism on Child and Adolescent Health." *Pediatrics* 144, no. 2 (August 1, 2019). https://doi.org/10.1542/peds.2019-1765.

Goyal, Monika K., Nathan Kuppermann, Sean D. Cleary, Stephen J. Teach, and James M. Chamberlain. "Racial Disparities in Pain Management of Children with Appendicitis in Emergency Departments." *JAMA Pediatrics* 169, no. 11 (November 1, 2015): 996–1002. https://doi.org/10.1001/jamapediatrics.2015.1915.

Brennan Ramirez, Laura K., Elizabeth A. Baker, and Marilyn Metzler. "Promoting Health Equity: A Resource to Help Communities Address Social Determinants of Health." *Department of Health and Human Services, Centers for Disease Control and Prevention*, January 1, 2008. https://www.cdc.gov/nccdphp/dch/programs/healthycommunitiesprogram/tools/pdf/sdoh-workbook.pdf.

Chantarat, Tongtan, David Van Riper, and Rachel R. Hardeman. "Multidimensional Structural Racism Predicts Birth Outcomes for Black and White Minnesotans." *Health Services Research* 57, no. 3 (April 25, 2022): 448–57. https://doi.org/10.1111/1475-6773.13976.

Geronimus, A. T. "The Weathering Hypothesis and the Health of African-American Women and Infants: Evidence and Speculations." *Ethnicity & Disease* 2, no. 3 (Summer 1992): 207–21. https://pubmed.ncbi.nlm.nih.gov/1467758/.

Forde, Allana T., Danielle M. Crookes, Shakira F. Suglia, and Ryan T. Demmer. "The Weathering Hypothesis as an Explanation for Racial Disparities in Health: A Systematic Review." *Annals of Epidemiology* 33 (May 1, 2019): 1–18.e3. https://doi.org/10.1016/j.annepidem.2019.02.011.

FFBWW. "Saving Our Babies: Low Birthweight Engagement Final Report." *The Foundation for Black Women's Wellness*, February 28, 2019.

Hardeman, Rachel R., Tongtan Chantarat, Morrison Luke Smith, J'Mag Karbeah, David Van Riper, and Dara D. Mendez. "Association of Residence in High-Police Contact Neighborhoods with Preterm Birth among Black and White Individuals in Minneapolis." *JAMA Network Open* 4, no. 12 (December 8, 2021): e2130290. https://doi.org/10.1001/jamanetworkopen.2021.30290.

Kappeler, Victor E. "A Brief History of Slavery and the Origins of American Policing." *EKU Online*, January 7, 2014. https://ekuonline.eku.edu/blog/police-studies/brief-history-slavery-and-origins-american-policing/.

Equal Justice Initiative. "Police Killings against Native Americans Are off the Charts and off the Radar," October 31, 2016. https://eji.org/news/native-americans-killed-by-police-at-highest-rate-in-country/.

Powell, Teran. "Native Americans Most Likely to Die from Police Shootings, Families Who Lost Loved Ones Weigh In." *WUWM 89.7 FM, Milwaukee's NPR*, June 2, 2021. https://www.wuwm.com/2021-06-02/native-americans-most-likely-to-die-from-police-shootings-families-who-lost-loved-ones-weigh-in.

"Rate of fatal police shootings in the United States from 2015 to October 2023, by ethnicity." *Statista*, September 5, 2023. https://www.statista.com/statistics/1123070/police-shootings-rate-ethnicity-us/.

"Angela Davis on the Argument for Police and Prison Abolition." Interview by Marc Hill, YouTube video. *Al Jazeera English*, December 17, 2021. https://www.youtube.com/watch?v=ZnRUHYkjwx4.

Hilal, Maha. *Innocent until Proven Muslim: Islamophobia, the War on Terror, and the Muslim Experience since 9/11.* Broadleaf Books, 2021.

Fraunfelder, Frederick T. "Is CS Gas Dangerous?" *The British Medical Journal* 320, no. 7233 (February 19, 2000): 458–59. https://doi.org/10.1136/bmj.320.7233.458.

Dowling, Jennifer. "Parents Again Decry Munitions Used by Feds near Cottonwood School." *Koin 6 News.* April 11, 2021. https://www.koin.com/news/protests/parents-decry-munitions-used-by-feds-near-cotton-wood-school/.

Beckett, Lois. "Teargas, Flash-Bangs: The Devastating Toll of Police Tactics on Minnesota Children." *The Guardian*, April 30, 2021. https://www.theguardian.com/us-news/2021/apr/30/teargas-effect-children-police-minnesota-brooklyn-center.

Critchfield, Hannah. "Pepper-sprayed on Their Way to the Polls: What Is Pepper Spray's Impact on Children?" *North Carolina Health News*, November 3, 2020. https://www.northcarolinahealthnews.org/2020/11/03/pepper-spray-more-dangerous-for-children-experts-say/.

Gordon, Scott. "Banning Tear Gas in Madison Shouldn't Even Be a Debate." *Tone Madison*, July 16, 2020. https://tonemadison.com/articles/banning-tear-gas-in-madison-shouldnt-even-be-a-debate/.

Schep, Leo J., Robin J. Slaughter, and David McBride. "Riot Control Agents: The Tear Gases CN, CS and OC—a Medical Review." *BMJ Military Health* 161, no. 2 (December 30, 2013): 94–99. https://doi.org/10.1136/jramc-2013-000165.

Arbak, Peri, Ilknur Baser, Özlem Ozdemir Kumbasar, Füsun Ülger, Zeki Kiliçaslan, and Fatma Evyapan. "Long Term Effects of Tear Gases on Respiratory System: Analysis of 93 Cases." *The Scientific World Journal* 2014 (January 1, 2014): 1–5. https://doi.org/10.1155/2014/963638.

Green, Tiffany, Jasmine Y. Zapata, Heidi W. Brown, and Nao Hagiwara. "Rethinking Bias to Achieve Maternal Health Equity: Changing Organizations, Not Just Individuals." *Obstetrics & Gynecology* 137, no. 5 (April 6, 2021): 935–40. https://doi.org/10.1097/aog.0000000000004363.

"Black Maternal Health Momnibus." *Black Maternal Health Caucus.* 2023. https://blackmaternalhealthcaucus-underwood.house.gov/Momnibus.

Vyas, Darshali A., Leo G. Eisenstein, and David S. Jones. "Hidden in Plain Sight—Reconsidering the Use of Race Correction in Clinical Algorithms." *The New England Journal of Medicine* 383, no. 9 (August 27, 2020): 874–82. https://doi.org/10.1056/nejmms2004740.

Rubashkin, Nicholas. "Why Equitable Access to Vaginal Birth Requires Abolition of Race-Based Medicine." *AMA Journal of Ethics* 24, no. 3 (March 1, 2022): E233–38. https://doi.org/10.1001/amajethics.2022.233.

Malat, Jennifer, Sarah Mayorga-Gallo, and David R. Williams. "The Effects of Whiteness on the Health of Whites in the USA." *Social Science & Medicine* 199 (February 1, 2018): 148–56. https://doi.org/10.1016/j.socscimed.2017.06.034.

Yearby, Ruqaiijah. "Race Based Medicine, Colorblind Disease: How Racism in Medicine Harms Us All." *The American Journal of Bioethics* 21, no. 2 (December 5, 2020): 19–27. https://doi.org/10.1080/15265161.2020.1851811.

Wang, Wen, Tracy L. Spinrad, Deborah Laible, Jayley Janssen, Sonya Xinyue Xiao, Jingyi Xu, Rebecca H. Berger, et al. "Parents' Color-Blind Racial Ideology and Implicit Racial Attitudes Predict Children's Race-Based Sympathy." *Journal of Family Psychology* 37, no. 4 (June 1, 2023): 475–85. https://doi.org/10.1037/fam0001047.

Garlinghouse, Rachel. "The Wildly Inappropriate Things People Ask Adoptive, Multiracial Families." *Tinybeans*, November 4, 2022. https://tinybeans.com/adoptive-multiracial-family-questions/.

Pratt, Beverly M., Lindsay Hixson, and Nicholas A. Jones. "Measuring Race and Ethnicity across the Decades: 1790–2010." *United States Census Bureau.* Accessed September 15, 2023. https://www.census.gov/data-tools/demo/race/MREAD_1790_2010.html.

Lewis, Anna, Santiago J. Molina, Paul S. Appelbaum, Bege Dauda, Anna Di Rienzo, Agustín Fuentes, Stephanie M. Fullerton, et al. "Getting Genetic Ancestry Right for Science and Society." *Science* 376, no. 6590 (April 14, 2022): 250–52. https://doi.org/10.1126/science.abm7530.

Ball, Philip. "Strangers Are Just Relatives You Haven't Met Yet." *Nature*, March 11, 1999. https://doi.org/10.1038/news990311-2.

Levey, Andrew S., Juan P. Bosch, Julia Breyer Lewis, Tom Greene, Nancy L. Rogers, and David Roth. "A More Accurate Method to Estimate Glomerular Filtration Rate from Serum Creatinine: A New Prediction Equation." *Annals of Internal Medicine* 130, no. 6 (March 16, 1999): 461. https://doi.org/10.7326/0003-4819-130-6-199903160-00002.

Tsai, Jennifer. "Jordan Crowley Would Be in Line for a Kidney—If He Were Deemed White Enough." *Slate*, June 27, 2021. https://slate.com/technology/2021/06/kidney-transplant-dialysis-race-adjustment.html.

CDC. "What Is Sickle Cell Disease?" *Centers for Disease Control and Prevention*. August 18, 2022. https://www.cdc.gov/ncbddd/sicklecell/facts.html.

Piel, Frédéric B., Anand P. Patil, Rosalind E. Howes, Oscar A. Nyangiri, Peter W. Gething, Thomas N. Williams, D. J. Weatherall, and Simon I. Hay. "Global Distribution of the Sickle Cell Gene and Geographical Confirmation of the Malaria Hypothesis." *Nature Communications* 1, no. 1 (November 2, 2010). https://doi.org/10.1038/ncomms1104.

Power-Hays, Alexandra, and Patrick T. McGann. "When Actions Speak Louder than Words—Racism and Sickle Cell Disease." *The New England Journal of Medicine* 383, no. 20 (November 12, 2020): 1902–03. https://doi.org/10.1056/nejmp2022125.

Harmon, Amy. "Can Biology Class Reduce Racism?" *The New York Times*, December 7, 2019. https://www.nytimes.com/2019/12/07/us/race-biology-genetics.html.

Kendi, Ibram X. *How to Raise an Antiracist*. One World, 2023.

Purnell, Tanjala S., Wanda Irving, Soleil Irving, Lauren Underwood, Raegan McDonald-Mosley, Chidinma A. Ibe, Debra L. Hickman, and Janice V. Bowie. "Honoring Dr. Shalon Irving, A Champion for Health Equity." *Health Affairs* 41, no. 2 (February 1, 2022): 304–08. https://doi.org/10.1377/hlthaff.2021.01447.

Naughton, Cynthia A. "Patient-Centered Communication." *Pharmacy* 6, no. 1 (February 13, 2018): 18. https://doi.org/10.3390/pharmacy6010018.

Sun, Michael, Tomasz Oliwa, Monica E. Peek, and Elizabeth L. Tung. "Negative Patient Descriptors: Documenting Racial Bias in the Electronic

Health Record." *Health Affairs* 41, no. 2 (January 19, 2022): 203–11. https://doi.org/10.1377/hlthaff.2021.01423.

5: case studies in parenting with feminism: bodily autonomy, ableism, and fatphobia

ACOG. "Assisted Vaginal Delivery: FAQs." *ACOG.* Accessed September 15, 2023. https://www.acog.org/womens-health/faqs/assisted-vaginal-delivery.

Betrán, Ana Pilar, Torloni, Jingfa Zhang, and A. Metin Gülmezoglu. "WHO Statement on Caesarean Section Rates." BJOG: An International Journal of Obstetrics and Gynaecology 123, no. 5 (July 22, 2015): 667–70. https://doi.org/10.1111/1471-0528.13526.

Taylor, Jamila K. "Structural Racism and Maternal Health among Black Women." *Journal of Law Medicine & Ethics* 48, no. 3 (January 1, 2020): 506–17. https://doi.org/10.1177/1073110520958875.

Larsson, Christina, Sissel Saltvedt, Ingela Wiklund, and Ellika Andolf. "Planned Vaginal Delivery versus Planned Caesarean Section: Short-Term Medical Outcome Analyzed According to Intended Mode of Delivery." *Journal of Obstetrics and Gynaecology Canada* 33, no. 8 (August 1, 2011): 796–802. https://doi.org/10.1016/s1701-2163(16)34982-9.

Committee on Obstetric Practice. "Cesarean Delivery on Maternal Request." *ACOG,* Committee Opinion no. 761. January 2019. https://www.acog.org/clinical/clinical-guidance/committee-opinion/articles/2019/01/cesarean-delivery-on-maternal-request.

Romanis, Elizabeth Chloe. "Why the Elective Caesarean Lottery Is Ethically Impermissible." *Health Care Analysis* 27, no. 4 (April 29, 2019): 249–68. https://doi.org/10.1007/s10728-019-00370-0.

Molina, George, Thomas Weiser, Stuart R. Lipsitz, Micaela Esquivel, Tarsicio Uribe-Leitz, Tej D. Azad, Neel Shah, et al. "Relationship between Cesarean Delivery Rate and Maternal and Neonatal Mortality." *JAMA* 314, no. 21 (December 1, 2015): 2263–70. https://doi.org/10.1001/jama.2015.15553.

Choate, Peter, and Christina Tortorelli. "Attachment Theory: A Barrier for Indigenous Children Involved with Child Protection." *International Journal of Environmental Research and Public Health* 19, no. 14 (July 19, 2022): 8754. https://doi.org/10.3390/ijerph19148754.

Chan, Katharine. "Why The Term 'Maternal Instinct' Hurts Men and Women." *An Injustice!,* April 17, 2020. https://aninjusticemag.com/why-the-term-maternal-instinct-hurts-men-and-women-e26489385520.

Young, Natalie A. E., and Katrina Crankshaw. "Disability Rates Highest among American Indian and Alaska Native Children and Children Living in Poverty." *United States Census Bureau*. October 8, 2021. https://www. census.gov/library/stories/2021/03/united-states-childhood-disability-rate-up-in-2019-from-2008.html.

CDC. "Disability Inclusion." *Centers for Disease Control and Prevention*. April 9, 2019. https://www.cdc.gov/ncbddd/disabilityandhealth/disability-inclusion.html#ref.

Kim, Julie. "Special Ed Shouldn't Be Separate: Isolating Kids from Their Peers Is Unjust." *The Atlantic*, March 6, 2023. https://www.theatlantic.com/family/archive/2023/03/kids-disabilities-special-education-school-inclusive-education/673276/.

"Students with Disabilities." *National Center for Education Statistics*. US Department of Education, Institute of Education Sciences. Accessed September 15, 2023. https://nces.ed.gov/programs/coe/pdf/2023/cgg_508.pdf.

Hogan, Andrew J. "Social and Medical Models of Disability and Mental Health: Evolution and Renewal." *Canadian Medical Association Journal* 191, no. 1 (January 6, 2019): E16–18. https://doi.org/10.1503/cmaj.181008.

Oliver, Mike. "The Social Model of Disability: Thirty Years On." *Disability & Society* 28, no. 7 (July 22, 2013): 1024–26. https://doi.org/10.1080/09687599.2013.818773.

Hamraie, Aimi. "Universal Design and the Problem of 'Post-Disability' Ideology." *Design and Culture* 8, no. 3 (August 19, 2016): 285–309. https://doi.org/10.1080/17547075.2016.1218714.

Pellicano, Elizabeth, and Jacquiline den Houting. "Annual Research Review: Shifting from 'Normal Science' to Neurodiversity in Autism Science." *Journal of Child Psychology and Psychiatry* 63, no. 4 (November 3, 2021): 381–96. https://doi.org/10.1111/jcpp.13534.

Sargent, Zoe, and Vikram K. Jaswal. "'It's Okay If You Flap Your Hands': Non-autistic Children Do Not Object to Individual Unconventional Behaviors Associated with Autism." *Social Development* 31, no. 4 (November, 2022): 1211–30. https://doi.org/10.1111/sode.12600.

The Partnership for Inclusive Disaster Strategies. "Opposition to Recent Ableist Remarks from CDC Director," January 12, 2022. https://disaster-strategies.org/wp-content/uploads/2022/01/Letter-to-Dr-Walensky-Accessible.pdf.

Samuel, Alexandra. "Happy Mother's Day: Kids' Screen Time Is a Feminist Issue." *JSTOR Daily*, May 2, 2016. https://daily.jstor.org/screentime-feminist-issue/.

Montgomery, Amanda; Collaboratory for Health Justice (2021). "Public Health Needs to Decouple Weight and Health." *University of Illinois at Chicago*. Educational resource. https://doi.org/10.25417/uic.16823341.v1

Tomiyama, A. Janet, Deborah Carr, Ellen M. Granberg, Brenda Major, Eric Robinson, Angelina R. Sutin, and Alexandra Brewis. "How and Why Weight Stigma Drives the Obesity 'Epidemic' and Harms Health." *BMC Medicine* 16, no. 1 (August 15, 2018). https://doi.org/10.1186/s12916-018-1116-5.

Eknoyan, Garabed. "Adolphe Quetelet (1796–1874)—The Average Man and Indices of Obesity." *Nephrology Dialysis Transplantation* 23, no. 1 (January, 2008: 47–51. https://doi.org/10.1093/ndt/gfm517.

Jacobs, Alexander E. "How Body Mass Index Compromises Care of Patients with Disabilities." *AMA Journal of Ethics* 25, no. 7 (July 1, 2023): E545–49. https://doi.org/10.1001/amajethics.2023.545.

NPR. "Fat Phobia and Its Racist Past and Present." *NPR Short Wave*, podcast episode. July 21, 2020. https://www.npr.org/2020/07/20/893006538/fat-phobia-and-its-racist-past-and-present.

Puhl, Rebecca M., and Chelsea A. Heuer. "Obesity Stigma: Important Considerations for Public Health." *American Journal of Public Health* 100, no. 6 (September 20, 2011): 1019–28. https://doi.org/10.2105/ajph.2009.159491.

CNN. "Who's Fat? New Definition Adopted." *CNN Interactive*. June 17, 1998. http://www.cnn.com/HEALTH/9806/17/weight.guidelines/.

Tsai, Jennifer, Jessica P. Cerdeña, Rohan Khazanchi, Edwin Lindo, Jasmine R. Marcelin, Aishwarya Rajagopalan, Raquel Sofia Sandoval, Andrea Westby, and Clarence C. Gravlee. "There Is No 'African American Physiology': The Fallacy of Racial Essentialism." *Journal of Internal Medicine* 288, no. 3 (August 17, 2020): 368–70. https://doi.org/10.1111/joim.13153.

Gower, Barbara A., and Lauren A. Fowler. "Obesity in African-Americans: The Role of Physiology." *Journal of Internal Medicine* 288, no. 3 (July 9, 2020): 295–304. https://doi.org/10.1111/joim.13090.

Gower, Barbara A., Lauren A. Fowler, and José R. Fernández. "Response to Tsai and Colleagues." *Journal of Internal Medicine* 288, no. 3 (August 3, 2020): 371–72. https://doi.org/10.1111/joim.13152.

Haqq, Andrea M., Maryam Kebbe, Qiming Tan, Melania Manco, and Ximena Ramos Salas. "Complexity and Stigma of Pediatric Obesity." *Childhood Obesity* 17, no. 4 (May 20, 2021): 229–40. https://doi.org/10.1089/chi.2021.0003.

Bodnar, Anastasia. "Internet Safety for Kids." *SciMoms*, May 6, 2019.

"Digital Citizenship Resources for Family Engagement." *Common Sense Education*. Accessed September 15, 2023. https://www.commonsense.org/education/family-resources.

"Beyond Screen Time: Help Your Kids Build Healthy Media Use Habits." *HealthyChildren.org*, 2022. Accessed September 15, 2023. https://www.healthychildren.org/English/family-life/Media/Pages/Healthy-Digital-Media-Use-Habits-for-Babies-Toddlers-Preschoolers.aspx.

"Beyond Screen Time: A Parent's Guide to Media Use." *AAP Publications, Pediatric Patient Education*, January 1, 2021. https://doi.org/10.1542/peo_document099.

"Health Advisory on Social Media Use in Adolescence." *American Psychological Association*, May 2023. https://www.apa.org/topics/social-media-internet/health-advisory-adolescent-social-media-use.

6: a clean life

Glassman, James K. "Dihydrogen Monoxide: Unrecognized Killer." *Washington Post*, October 21, 1997.

Cantrill, Stuart. "A Chemical-Free Paper." *The Sceptical Chymist—A Blog from Nature Chemistry*, June 26, 2014. Accessed September 16, 2023. https://blogs.nature.com/thescepticalchymist/2014/06/a-chemical-free-paper.html.

"Public Attitudes to Chemistry." Research Report. *Royal Society of Chemistry*, 2015. https://www.rsc.org/policy-evidence-campaigns/outreach/public-attitudes-chemistry/.

Lorch, Mark. "Chemophobia, a Chemists' Construct." *Royal Society of Chemistry*, July 2015. https://www.rsc.org/news-events/opinions/2015/jul/chemophobia-mark-lorch/.

USDA. "Dietary Guidelines for Americans 2020–2025." *US Departments of Agriculture and Health and Human Services*, 2020. https://www.dietaryguidelines.gov/sites/default/files/2021-03/Dietary_Guidelines_for_Americans-2020-2025.pdf.

Kell, John. "Panera Says Its Food Menu Is Now 100% 'Clean Eating.'" *Fortune*, January 13, 2017. https://fortune.com/2017/01/13/panera-menu-completely-clean/.

Geha, Raif S., Alexa S. Beiser, Clement L. Ren, Roy Patterson, Paul A. Greenberger, Leslie C. Grammer, Anne Marie Ditto, et al. "Review of Alleged Reaction to Monosodium Glutamate and Outcome of a Multi-center Double-Blind Placebo-Controlled Study." *Journal of Nutrition* 130, no. 4 (April 1, 2000): 1058S–62S. https://doi.org/10.1093/jn/130.4.1058s.

Bernstein, Alison, and Iida Ruishalme. "Risk in Perspective." *SciMoms*, February 22, 2018.

"Family Eats Organic for Just Two Weeks, Removes Nearly All Pesticides from Body," *Sydney Morning Herald*, May 13, 2015. https://www.smh.com.au/lifestyle/health-and-wellness/family-eats-organic-for-just-two-weeks-removes-nearly-all-pesticides-from-body-20150513-gh0jhd.html.

Mallon, Melanie. "Bad Chart Thursday: Organic Cherry Picking." *Skepchick*, May 18, 2015. https://skepchick.org/2015/05/bad-chart-thursday-organic-cherry-picking/.

Bernstein, Alison. "Defining Safety: How Safe Is Safe?" *SciMoms*, April 26, 2018.

Caron, Christina. "Why Do Parents Keep Hearing about the Microbiome?" *The New York Times*, October 17, 2019. https://www.nytimes.com/2021/07/25/parenting/baby/microbiome-health.html.

Eisen, Jonathan A. "Microbiomania." *The Tree of Life* (blog), June 19, 2014. Accessed September 16, 2023. https://phylogenomics.blogspot.com/p/blog-page.html.

Center on the Developing Child. "What Is Epigenetics? How Children's Experiences Affect Their Genes." *Harvard University*, October 30, 2020. https://developingchild.harvard.edu/resources/what-is-epigenetics-and-how-does-it-relate-to-child-development/.

Blaze, Jennifer, and Tania L. Roth. "Evidence from Clinical and Animal Model Studies of the Long-Term and Transgenerational Impact of Stress on DNA Methylation." *Seminars in Cell & Developmental Biology* 43 (July 1, 2015): 76–84. https://doi.org/10.1016/j.semcdb.2015.04.004.

CDC. "Antibiotic Do's & Don'ts" *Centers for Disease Control and Prevention.* Accessed September 16, 2023. https://www.cdc.gov/antibiotic-use/do-and-dont.html.

Alison Bernstein and Iida Ruishalme. "Risk in Perspective: Population Risk Does Not Equal Individual Risk," *SciMoms,* April 4, 2018.

Coggon, D., Geoffrey Rose, and D.J.P. Barker. "Chapter 1. What Is Epidemiology?" In *Epidemiology for the Uninitiated,* Fourth Edition. BMJ Books, 1997. https://www.bmj.com/about-bmj/resources-readers/publications/epidemiology-uninitiated/1-what-epidemiology.

Cook, Lola, Jeanine Schulze, Wendy R. Uhlmann, Jennifer Verbrugge, Karen Marder, Annie J. Lee, Yuanjia Wang, Roy N. Alcalay, Martha Nance, and James C. Beck. "Tools for Communicating Risk for Parkinson's Disease." *npj Parkinson's Disease* 8, no. 1 (November 29, 2022). https://doi.org/10.1038/s41531-022-00432-6.

CBS News. "Chemical Linked to Cancer Found in Breakfast Foods." *CBS News,* August 15, 2018. https://www.cbsnews.com/video/chemical-linked-to-cancer-found-in-breakfast-foods/.

Mesnage, Robin, and Michael Antoniou. "Facts and Fallacies in the Debate on Glyphosate Toxicity." *Frontiers in Public Health* 5 (November 24, 2017). https://doi.org/10.3389/fpubh.2017.00316.

Tarone, Robert E. "On the International Agency for Research on Cancer Classification of Glyphosate as a Probable Human Carcinogen." *European Journal of Cancer Prevention* 27, no. 1 (January 1, 2018): 82–87. https://doi.org/10.1097/cej.0000000000000289.

Canadian Centre for Occupational Health and Safety. "What Is a LD50 and LC50?" *Government of Canada,* June 13, 2023. https://www.ccohs.ca/oshanswers/chemicals/ld50.html.

Zbinden, G., and M. Flury-Roversi. "Significance of the LD50-Test for the Toxicological Evaluation of Chemical Substances." *Archives of Toxicology* 47, no. 2 (April 1, 1981): 77–99. https://doi.org/10.1007/bf00332351.

Brunning, Andy. "Lethal Doses of Water, Caffeine and Alcohol." *Compound Interest,* July 27, 2014. https://www.compoundchem.com/2014/07/27/lethaldoses/.

Katiraee, Layla. "Is Caffeine Safe for Children?" *SciMoms,* July 9, 2019.

Ruishalme, Iida, and Alison Bernstein. "Measures of Toxicity." *Thoughtscapism* (blog), May 7, 2018. https://thoughtscapism.com/2018/05/07/measures-of-toxicity/.

CBC. "Man Treated for Cyanide Poisoning from Apricot Kernels Says, 'Selling Them like Nuts Is Nuts.'" *As It Happens*, CBC Radio, November 24, 2017. https://www.cbc.ca/radio/asithappens/as-it-happens-friday-edition-1.4417898/man-treated-for-cyanide-poisoning-from-apricot-kernels-says-selling-them-like-nuts-is-nuts-1.4417904.

US EPA. "Reference Dose (RfD): Description and Use in Health Risk Assessments, Background Document 1A." *United States Environmental Protection Agency.* March 15, 1993. Accessed September 16, 2023. https://www.epa.gov/iris/reference-dose-rfd-description-and-use-health-risk-assessments.

Kanissery, Ramdas, Biwek Gairhe, Davie M. Kadyampakeni, Ozgur Batuman, and Fernando Alferez. "Glyphosate: Its Environmental Persistence and Impact on Crop Health and Nutrition." *Plants* 8, no. 11 (November 13, 2019): 499. https://doi.org/10.3390/plants8110499.

EWG. "Roundup for Breakfast, Part 2: In New Tests, Weed Killer Found in All Kids' Cereals Sampled." *Environmental Working Group*, October 24, 2018. https://www.ewg.org/news-insights/news-release/2018/10/roundup-breakfast-part-2-new-tests-weed-killer-found-all-kids.

Matthews, Susan. "You Don't Need to Worry about Roundup in Your Breakfast Cereal." *Slate*, August 16, 2018. https://slate.com/technology/2018/08/glyphosate-from-monsantos-weed-killer-roundup-in-breakfast-cereal-isnt-something-to-worry-about.html.

Gilmer, Marcus. "Don't Worry, Your Cereal Probably Won't Poison You with Pesticides." *Mashable*, August 17, 2018. https://mashable.com/article/cereal-glyphosate-pesticide-study-debunk.

IARC. "Agents Classified by the IARC Monographs, Volumes 1–134," IARC Monographs on the Identification of Carcinogenic Hazards to Humans, *World Health Organization.* n.d. https://monographs.iarc.who.int/agents-classified-by-the-iarc/.

US EPA. "Evaluating Pesticides for Carcinogenic Potential." *United States Environmental Protection Agency.* June 30, 2023. https://www.epa.gov/pesticide-science-and-assessing-pesticide-risks/evaluating-pesticides-carcinogenic-potential.

Yong, Ed. "Beefing With the World Health Organization's Cancer Warnings" *The Atlantic*, October 26, 2015. https://www.theatlantic.com/health/archive/2015/10/why-is-the-world-health-organization-so-bad-at-communicating-cancer-risk/412468/.

US EPA. "Health Risk of Radon." *United States Environmental Protection Agency*. January 5, 2023. https://www.epa.gov/radon/health-risk-radon.

Wisconsin Department of Health Services. "Lowering Your Home's Radon Levels." July 20, 2023. https://www.dhs.wisconsin.gov/radon/reduce-radon.htm.

Rabbitt, Matthew P., Alisha Coleman-Jensen, and Christian A. Gregory. "Understanding the Prevalence, Severity, and Distribution of Food Insecurity in the United States." *USDA Economic Research Service*. September 6, 2017. https://www.ers.usda.gov/amber-waves/2017/september/understanding-the-prevalence-severity-and-distribution-of-food-insecurity-in-the-united-states/.

Dahmer, David. "Food Desert No More: Luna's Groceries Officially Open for Business." *Madison365*, January 29, 2019. https://madison365.com/food-desert-no-more-lunas-groceries-officially-open-for-business/.

States, Joe, and Lauryn Azu. "Wisconsin: Land of Plenty Includes Plenty of 'Food Deserts': Large Parts of Milwaukee and Rural Wisconsin Lack Easy Access to Groceries. The State, Cities and Communities Are Working to Change That." *Wisconsin Watch*, September 1, 2022. https://wisconsinwatch.org/2022/09/wisconsin-land-of-plenty-includes-plenty-of-food-deserts/.

"Urban Growers Collective: Cultivating Pathways to Freedom through Food & Healing." Urban Growers Collective. Accessed September 16, 2023. https://www.urbangrowerscollective.org/.

Zeratsky, Katherine. On Whether Phenylalanine in Diet Soda Is Harmful. *Expert Answers, Mayo Clinic*. Accessed September 16, 2023. https://www.mayoclinic.org/healthy-lifestyle/nutrition-and-healthy-eating/expert-answers/phenylalanine/faq-20058361.

Abrams, Steven A. "Is Homemade Baby Formula Safe?" *HealthyChildren.org*. Accessed September 16, 2023. https://www.healthychildren.org/English/ages-stages/baby/formula-feeding/Pages/Is-Homemade-Baby-Formula-Safe.aspx.

NHS. "Homeopathy," February 22, 2022. NHS. Accessed September 16, 2023. https://www.nhs.uk/conditions/homeopathy/.

"How to Care for Your Child's Cold." *HealthyChildren.org*. Accessed September 16, 2023. https://www.healthychildren.org/English/health-issues/conditions/flu/Pages/caring-for-Your-childs-cold-or-flu.aspx.

Bodnar, Anastasia. "Safe Teething Remedies." *SciMoms*, July 3, 2021.

US FDA. "Safely Soothing Teething Pain and Sensory Needs in Babies and Older Children." US Food and Drug Administration. 2018. Accessed September 16, 2023. https://www.fda.gov/consumers/consumer-updates/safely-soothing-teething-pain-and-sensory-needs-babies-and-older-children.

Grelotti, David J., and Ted J. Kaptchuk. "Placebo by Proxy." *BMJ* 343 (August 11, 2011): d4345. https://doi.org/10.1136/bmj.d4345.

US EPA. "Learn about Lead." *United States Environmental Protection Agency*. August 28, 2023. https://www.epa.gov/lead/learn-about-lead.

McFarland, Michael J., Mathew Hauer, and Aaron Reuben. "Half of US Population Exposed to Adverse Lead Levels in Early Childhood." *PNAS* 119, no. 11 (March 7, 2022). https://doi.org/10.1073/pnas.2118631119.

Kennedy, Merrit. "Lead-Laced Water in Flint: A Step-By-Step Look at the Makings of a Crisis." *NPR*, April 20, 2016. https://www.npr.org/sections/thetwo-way/2016/04/20/465545378/lead-laced-water-in-flint-a-step-by-step-look-at-the-makings-of-a-crisis.

US EPA. "EPA Releases First-Ever Agency-Wide Strategy to Reduce Lead Exposures and Disparities in US Communities." *United States Environmental Protection Agency*. October 27, 2022. https://www.epa.gov/newsreleases/epa-releases-first-ever-agency-wide-strategy-reduce-lead-exposures-and-disparities-us.

Susan Selasky. "Fight Lead Exposure with Nutrient-Rich Foods." *Detroit Free Press*, February 4, 2016. https://www.freep.com/story/life/food/recipes/2016/02/04/nutrion-lead-fighting-foods/79838898/.

US EPA. "Our Current Understanding of the Human Health and Environmental Risks of PFAS." *United States Environmental Protection Agency*. June 7, 2023. https://www.epa.gov/pfas/our-current-understanding-human-health-and-environmental-risks-pfas.

ATSDR. "What Are the Health Effects of PFAS?" Agency for Toxic Substances and Disease Registry. Accessed September 16, 2023. https://www.atsdr.cdc.gov/pfas/health-effects/index.html.

Kwiatkowski, Carol F., David Q. Andrews, Linda S. Birnbaum, Thomas A. Bruton, Jamie C. DeWitt, Detlef R. U. Knappe, Maricel V. Maffini, et al. "Scientific Basis for Managing PFAS as a Chemical Class." *Environmental Science and Technology Letters* 7, no. 8 (June 30, 2020): 532–43. https://doi.org/10.1021/acs.estlett.0c00255.

Maertens, Alexandra, Emily Golden, and Thomas Hartung. "Avoiding Regrettable Substitutions: Green Toxicology for Sustainable Chemistry." *ACS Sustainable Chemistry & Engineering* 9, no. 23 (June 1, 2021): 7749–58. https://doi.org/10.1021/acssuschemeng.0c09435.

Cousins, Ian T., Jana H. Johansson, Matthew Salter, Bo Sha, and Martin Scheringer. "Outside the Safe Operating Space of a New Planetary Boundary for Per- and Polyfluoroalkyl Substances (PFAS)." *Environmental Science & Technology* 56, no. 16 (August 2, 2022): 11172–179. https://doi.org/10.1021/acs.est.2c02765.

US EPA. "Meaningful and Achievable Steps You Can Take to Reduce Your Risk." *United States Environmental Protection Agency.* August 8, 2023. https://www.epa.gov/pfas/meaningful-and-achievable-steps-you-can-take-reduce-your-risk.

Babrauskas, Vytenis, Arlene Blum, R. D. Daley, and Linda S. Birnbaum. "Flame Retardants in Furniture Foam: Benefits and Risks." *Fire Safety Science* 10 (January 1, 2011): 265–78. https://doi.org/10.3801/iafss.fss.10-265.

"PBBs (Polybrominated Biphenyls) in Michigan : Frequently Asked Questions, 2011 Update." *Michigan Department of Community Health.* https://www.michigan.gov/-/media/Project/Websites/mdhhs/Folder1/Folder26/mdch_PBB_FAQ.pdf.

7: greenwashing our children's future

Zipper, David. "The Unstoppable Appeal of Highway Expansion." *Bloomberg*, September 28, 2021. https://www.bloomberg.com/news/features/2021-09-28/why-widening-highways-doesn-t-bring-traffic-relief.

Mann, Denise. "Move to 'Zero-Emission' Vehicles Would Save 90,000 US Lives by 2050." *US News & World Report*, June 7, 2023. https://www.usnews.com/news/health-news/articles/2023-06-07/move-to-zero-emission-vehicles-would-save-90-000-u-s-lives-by-2050.

Taylor, Nandi L., Jamila M. Porter, Shenee J. Bryan, Katherine J. Harmon, and Laura Sandt. "Structural Racism and Pedestrian Safety: Measuring the Association between Historical Redlining and Contemporary Pedestrian Fatalities across the United States, 2010-2019." *American Journal of Public Health* 113, no. 4 (April 1, 2023): 420–28. https://doi.org/10.2105/ajph. 2022.307192.

"What Is the Carbon Cycle?" *National Ocean Service, National Oceanic and Atmospheric Administration.* Accessed September 16, 2023. https://oceanservice. noaa.gov/facts/carbon-cycle.html.

Buis, Alan. "Steamy Relationships: How Atmospheric Water Vapor Amplifies Earth's Greenhouse Effect." *Climate Change: Vital Signs of the Planet* (blog), February 8, 2022. https://climate.nasa.gov/explore/ask-nasa-climate/3143/ steamy-relationships-how-atmospheric-water-vapor-amplifies-earths-green-house-effect/.

Thulin, Lila. "How an Oil Spill Inspired the First Earth Day." *Smithsonian Magazine*, April 22, 2019. https://www.smithsonianmag.com/history/how-oil-spill-50-years-ago-inspired-first-earth-day-180972007/.

Green, K. C. "On Fire." *Gunshow* (comic), 2013. http://gunshowcomic.com/ 648.

Heglar, Mary Annaïse. "Climate Grief Hurts Because It's Supposed To." *The Nation*, November 7, 2021. https://www.thenation.com/article/ environment/climate-grief-hope/.

Splitter, Jenny. "Yes, You Should Still Reduce Your Personal Carbon Footprint: We Need to Hold Polluting Companies Accountable AND Eat Less Meat. Both Are Also Critical for Curbing Climate Change." *FutureFeed*, January 27, 2022. https://futurefeed.substack.com/p/yes-you-should-still-reduce-your.

Trembath, Alex, and Vijaya Ramachandran. "The Malthusians Are Back." *The Atlantic*, March 22, 2023. https://www.theatlantic.com/ideas/ archive/2023/03/population-control-movement-climate-malthusian-similarities/673450/.

"One Billion Children at 'Extremely High Risk' of the Impacts of the Climate Crisis." *UNICEF* (press release). August 19, 2021. https://www. unicef.org/press-releases/one-billion-children-extremely-high-risk-impacts-climate-crisis-unicef.

Chapman, Audrey R., and A. Karim Ahmed. "Climate Justice, Humans

Rights, and the Case for Reparations." *Health and Human Rights* 23, no. 2, December 1, 2021: 81–94. https://www.ncbi.nlm.nih.gov/pmc/articles/PMC8694300/.

MacGuire, Frances. "Climate Action for Health: COP27 Delivers on Reparation but Not Mitigation." *OECD Forum Network*, December 23, 2022. https://www.oecd-forum.org/posts/climate-action-for-health-cop27-delivers-on-reparation-but-not-mitigation.

Manann Donoghoe and Perry, Andre M. "The Case for Climate Reparations in the United States | Brookings." Brookings, March, 2023. https://www.brookings.edu/articles/the-case-for-climate-reparations-in-the-united-states/.

Watkins, Shannon Lea, and Ed Gerrish. "The Relationship between Urban Forests and Race: A Meta-analysis." *Journal of Environmental Management* 209 (March 1, 2018): 152–68. https://doi.org/10.1016/j.jenvman.2017.12.021.

Rockström, Johan, Joyeeta Gupta, Dahe Qin, Steven J. Lade, Jesse F. Abrams, Lauren S. Andersen, David I. Armstrong McKay, et al. "Safe and Just Earth System Boundaries." *Nature* 619, no. 7968 (May 31, 2023): 102–11. https://doi.org/10.1038/s41586-023-06083-8.

Khan, Andy And Ayesha. "Climate or Ecology?—The Gastropocene, Chapter II." *Cosmic Anarchy* (blog), November 2, 2022. https://wokescientist.substack.com/p/climate-or-ecology-the-gastropocene.

Walker, Erica D., Nina F. Lee, Koen F. Tieskens, Jonathan Jay, Lorrie J. Walker, Marisa Luse, Roudnie Celestin, Jerome Robert Smith, Julia Mejia, and Jonathan I. Levy. "Firework Activity and Environmental Sound Levels: Community Impacts and Solutions." *Cities & Health* 6, no. 3 (June 8, 2021): 552–63. https://doi.org/10.1080/23748834.2021.1928857.

NPR. "Fighting Noise Pollution." *Consider This, NPR* (podcast episode), August 18, 2023. https://www.npr.org/transcripts/1194676625.

The Associated Press. "The US Is Divided over Whether Nuclear Power Is Part of the Green Energy Future." *NPR*, January 18, 2022. https://www.npr.org/2022/01/18/1073726137/the-us-is-divided-over-whether-nuclear-power-is-part-of-the-green-energy-future.

Adams, Jarret. "Electric Vehicles Aren't Always Carbon-Free, But with Nuclear They Can Be." *Nuclear Energy Institute* (blog), April 10, 2019. https://www.nei.org/news/2019/electric-vehicles-carbon-free-nuclear-can-be.

Ritchie, Hannah. "What Are the Safest and Cleanest Sources of Energy?" *Our World in Data*, February 10, 2020. https://ourworldindata.org/safest-sources-of-energy.

Mothers for Nuclear. "Mothers for Nuclear." Accessed September 17, 2023. https://www.mothersfornuclear.org/.

Wang, Irina. "10 Years Ago, We Were Turning Nuclear Bombs into Nuclear Energy. We can do it again." *Vox*, February 14, 2023. https://www.vox.com/future-perfect/23593348/build-nuclear-energy-from-nuclear-bombs-ukraine-war.

Desai, Sheil. "Mining Indigenous Communities: A Long Legacy." *Kleinman Center for Energy Policy.* December 20, 2021. https://kleinmanenergy.upenn.edu/news-insights/mining-indigenous-communities-a-long-legacy/.

Office of Energy Efficiency and Renewable Energy. "Solar Integration: Solar Energy and Storage Basics." *United States Department of Energy.* Accessed September 17, 2023. https://www.energy.gov/eere/solar/solar-integration-solar-energy-and-storage-basics.

Heath, Joe. "The Violence of Nuclear Energy against Indigenous Peoples, Land, Water and Air." *Syracuse Peace Council's Peace Newsletter*, no. 871, March/April 2020: 8. https://peacecouncil.net/wp-content/uploads/2020/03/March_April-871-v14-FINAL-Color-photos.pdf.

Dowling, Jacqueline A., Katherine Z. Rinaldi, T. Ruggles, Steven J. Davis, Mengyao Yuan, Fan Tong, Nathan S. Lewis, and Ken Caldeira. "Role of Long-Duration Energy Storage in Variable Renewable Electricity Systems." *Joule* 4, no. 9 (September 16, 2020): 1907–28. https://doi.org/10.1016/j.joule.2020.07.007.

Gutierrez, Grant. "We Must Take Care to Not 'Greenwash' Environmental Justice." *South Seattle Emerald*, May 8, 2023. https://southseattleemerald.com/2023/05/08/opinion-we-must-take-care-to-not-greenwash-environmental-justice/.

Obura, David, Fabrice DeClerck, P. H. Verburg, Joyeeta Gupta, Jesse F. Abrams, Xuemei Bai, Stuart Bunn, et al. "Achieving a Nature- and People-positive Future." *One Earth* 6, no. 2 (February 17, 2023): 105–17. https://doi.org/10.1016/j.oneear.2022.11.013.

De Freitas Netto, Sebastião Vieira, Marcos Felipe Falcão Sobral, Ana Regina Bezerra Ribeiro, and Gleibson Robert da Luz Soares. "Concepts and Forms of Greenwashing: A Systematic Review." *Environmental Sciences Europe* 32, no. 19 (February 11, 2020). https://doi.org/10.1186/s12302-020-0300-3.

Montgomery, A. Wren, Thomas P. Lyon, and Julian Barg. "No End in Sight? A Greenwash Review and Research Agenda." *Organization & Environment*, May 9, 2023, 108602662311689. https://doi.org/10.1177/10860266231168905.

Fulton, Kari. "Kari Fulton Looks Out for Greenwashing." *Big Think* (video), September 30, 2021. https://bigthink.com/videos/kari-fulton-looks-out-for-greenwashing/.

Heglar, Mary Annaïse. "Confessions of a Green Troll: On the Pleasures of Cyberbullying Oil Companies." *Orion Magazine*. Accessed September 17, 2023. https://orionmagazine.org/article/confessions-of-a-green-troll/.

BP. "The first step to reducing your emissions is to know where you stand…" *Twitter* (post), October 22, 2019. https://twitter.com/bp_plc/status/1186645440621531136.

smith, s. e. "Banning Straws Might Be a Win for Environmentalists. But It Ignores Us Disabled People." *Vox*, July 19, 2018. https://www.vox.com/first-person/2018/7/19/17587676/straws-plastic-ban-disability.

IUCN. "Issues Brief: Marine Plastic Pollution." *International Union for Conservation of Nature and Natural Resources*. November 2021. https://www.iucn.org/resources/issues-brief/marine-plastic-pollution.

Purkiss, Danielle, Ayse Lisa Allison, Fabiana Lorencatto, Susan Michie, and Mark Miodownik. "The Big Compost Experiment: Using Citizen Science to Assess the Impact and Effectiveness of Biodegradable and Compostable Plastics in UK Home Composting." *Frontiers in Sustainability* 3 (November 3, 2022). https://doi.org/10.3389/frsus.2022.942724.

Zhu, Jingkun, and Can Wang. "Biodegradable Plastics: Green Hope or Greenwashing?" *Marine Pollution Bulletin* 161, part B (December 1, 2020): 111774. https://doi.org/10.1016/j.marpolbul.2020.111774.

Heiges, Jessica, and Kate O'Neill. "What Is Wishcycling? Two Waste Experts Explain." *The Conversation*, January 12, 2022. https://theconversation.com/what-is-wishcycling-two-waste-experts-explain-173825.

UNEP. "Turning off the Tap: How the World Can End Plastic Pollution and Create a Circular Economy." *UN Environment Programme*. May 16, 2023. https://www.unep.org/resources/turning-off-tap-end-plastic-pollution-create-circular-economy.

United Nations. "Actions for a Healthy Planet." Accessed September 17, 2023. https://www.un.org/en/actnow/ten-actions.

Li, Mengyu, Nanfei Jia, Manfred Lenzen, Arunima Malik, Liyuan Wei, Yutong Jin, and David Raubenheimer. "Global Food-Miles Account for Nearly 20% of Total Food-Systems Emissions." *Nature Food* 3, no. 6 (June 20, 2022): 445–53. https://doi.org/10.1038/s43016-022-00531-w.

Nowell, Cecilia. "Is Eating Local Produce Actually Better for the Planet?" *The Guardian*, June 7, 2023. https://www.theguardian.com/environment/2023/jun/07/is-eating-local-better-environment.

"The Problem with Avocados." *Food Empowerment Project.* September 22, 2022. https://foodispower.org/our-food-choices/the-problem-with-avocados/.

Cho, Kimin, Benjamin Goldstein, Dimitrios Gounaridis, and Joshua P. Newell. "Where Does Your Guacamole Come From? Detecting Deforestation Associated with the Export of Avocados from Mexico to the United States." *Journal of Environmental Management* 278, part 1 (January 15, 2021): 111482. https://doi.org/10.1016/j.jenvman.2020.111482.

US EPA. "Report on the Environment: Land Use." *United States Environmental Protection Agency.* July 2023. Accessed September 17, 2023. https://www.epa.gov/report-environment/land-use.

FAO UN. "Land Use in Agriculture by the Numbers." *Food and Agriculture Organization of the United Nations.* May 7, 2020. https://www.fao.org/sustainability/news/detail/en/c/1274219/.

"Protein Scorecard." *World Resources Institute.* April 20, 2016. https://www.wri.org/data/protein-scorecard.

Ritchie, Hannah. "If the World Adopted a Plant-Based Diet We Would Reduce Global Agricultural Land Use from 4 to 1 Billion Hectares." *Our World in Data*, March 4, 2021. https://ourworldindata.org/land-use-diets.

Waite, Richard, Tim Searchinger, Janet Ranganathan, and Jessica Zionts. "6 Pressing Questions about Beef and Climate Change, Answered." *World Resources Institute.* March 7, 2022. Accessed September 17, 2023. https://www.wri.org/insights/6-pressing-questions-about-beef-and-climate-change-answered.

USDA. "Food Product Dating." *Food Safety and Inspection Service, USDA.* 2019. Accessed September 17, 2023. https://www.fsis.usda.gov/food-safety/safe-food-handling-and-preparation/food-safety-basics/food-product-dating.

Splitter, Jenny. "What Is the Best Milk for the Environment?" *SciMoms*, February 13, 2021.

Lebel, Eric D., Colin J Finnegan, Zutao Ouyang, and Robert B. Jackson. "Methane and NOx Emissions from Natural Gas Stoves, Cooktops, and Ovens in Residential Homes." *Environmental Science & Technology* 56, no. 4 (January 27, 2022): 2529–39. https://doi.org/10.1021/acs.est.1c04707.

Lewis, Tanya. "The Health Risks of Gas Stoves Explained." *Scientific American*. January 19, 2023. https://www.scientificamerican.com/article/the-health-risks-of-gas-stoves-explained/.

Shahmohammadi, Sadegh, Z.J.N. Steinmann, Lau Tambjerg, Patricia van Loon, Joseph M. Henry King, and Mark A. J. Huijbregts. "Comparative Greenhouse Gas Footprinting of Online versus Traditional Shopping for Fast-Moving Consumer Goods: A Stochastic Approach." *Environmental Science & Technology* 54, no. 6 (February 26, 2020): 3499–3509. https://doi.org/10.1021/acs.est.9b06252.

Heffernan, Tim. "How to Shop Online More Sustainably." *Wirecutter*, April 22, 2021. https://www.nytimes.com/wirecutter/blog/shop-online-sustainably/.

Bigazzi, Alexander. "Comparison of Marginal and Average Emission Factors for Passenger Transportation Modes." *Applied Energy* 242 (May 15, 2019): 1460–66. https://doi.org/10.1016/j.apenergy.2019.03.172.

Capehart, Tom, and Susan Proper. "Corn Is America's Largest Crop in 2019." *US Department of Agriculture.* July 29, 2019. https://www.usda.gov/media/blog/2019/07/29/corn-americas-largest-crop-2019.

Domel, Jessica. "5 Differences between Field Corn, Sweet Corn." *Texas Table Top, Texas Farm Bureau*, September 4, 2018. Accessed September 18, 2023. https://tabletop.texasfarmbureau.org/2018/09/5-differences-field-corn-sweet-corn/.

USDA Office of Communications. "USDA Coexistence Fact Sheets: Corn." *US Department of Agriculture*, press release, February 2015. https://www.usda.gov/sites/default/files/documents/coexistence-corn-factsheet.pdf.

Wang, Michael, Uisung Lee, Hoyoung Kwon, and Hui Xu. "Life-Cycle Greenhouse Gas Emission Reductions of Ethanol with the GREET Model." *Argonne National Laboratory*, February 17, 2021. https://afdc.energy.gov/files/u/publication/ethanol-ghg-reduction-with-greet.pdf.

Pellegrino, Elisa, Stefano Bedini, Marco Nuti, and Laura Ercoli. "Impact of Genetically Engineered Maize on Agronomic, Environmental and Toxicological Traits: A Meta-analysis of 21 Years of Field Data." *Scientific Reports* 8, no. 1 (February 15, 2018). https://doi.org/10.1038/s41598-018-21284-2.

Prokopy, Linda Stalker, Benjamin M. Gramig, Alisha Bower, Sarah P. Church, Brenna Ellison, Philip W. Gassman, Ken Genskow, et al. "The Urgency of Transforming the Midwestern US Landscape into More Than Corn and Soybean." *Agriculture and Human Values* 37, no. 3 (May 23, 2020): 537–39. https://doi.org/10.1007/s10460-020-10077-x.

Holland, Austin, David A. Bennett, and Silvia Secchi. "Complying with Conservation Compliance? An Assessment of Recent Evidence in the US Corn Belt." *Environmental Research Letters* 15, no. 8 (August 7, 2020): 084035. https://doi.org/10.1088/1748-9326/ab8f60.

Siegel, Karen R., Kai McKeever Bullard, Giuseppina Imperatore, Henry S. Kahn, Aryeh D. Stein, Mohammed K. Ali, and K. M. Venkat Narayan. "Association of Higher Consumption of Foods Derived from Subsidized Commodities with Adverse Cardiometabolic Risk among US Adults." *JAMA Internal Medicine* 176, no. 8 (August 1, 2016): 1124. https://doi.org/10.1001/jamainternmed.2016.2410.

8: vaccines

CDC. "Fast Facts on Global Immunization." *Centers for Disease Control and Prevention*. April 20, 2023. Accessed September 18, 2023. https://www.cdc.gov/globalhealth/immunization/data/fast-facts.html.

WHO. "Vaccine-Preventable Diseases (including Pipeline Vaccines)." *Immunization, Vaccines and Biologicals Department, World Health Organization*. Accessed September 18, 2023. https://www.who.int/teams/immunization-vaccines-and-biologicals/diseases.

Pollard, Andrew J., and Else M. Bijker. "A Guide to Vaccinology: From Basic Principles to New Developments." *Nature Reviews Immunology* 21, no. 2 (December 22, 2020): 83–100. https://doi.org/10.1038/s41577-020-00479-7.

Netea, Mihai G., Jorge Domínguez-Andrés, Luis B. Barreiro, Triantafyllos Chavakis, Maziar Divangahi, Elaine Fuchs, Leo A. B. Joosten, et al. "Defining Trained Immunity and Its Role in Health and Disease." *Nature Reviews Immunology* 20, no. 6 (March 4, 2020): 375–88. https://doi.org/10.1038/s41577-020-0285-6.

Durrheim, David N. "Measles Eradication—Retreating Is Not an Option." *The Lancet, Infectious Diseases* 20, no. 6 (March 17, 2020): e138–41. https://doi.org/10.1016/s1473-3099(20)30052-9.

Yang, Luojun, Bryan T. Grenfell, and Michael J. Mina. "Waning Immunity and Re-emergence of Measles and Mumps in the Vaccine Era." *Current *Opinion in Virology* 40 (February 1, 2020): 48–54. https://doi.org/10.1016/ j.coviro.2020.05.009.

CDC. "Explaining How Vaccines Work." *Centers for Disease Control and Prevention.* May 24, 2023. Accessed September 18, 2023. https://www.cdc.gov/ vaccines/hcp/conversations/understanding-vacc-work.html.

Smith, Tara C. "Vaccine Rejection and Hesitancy: A Review and Call to Action." *Open Forum Infectious Diseases* 4, no. 3 (Summer, 2017). https:// doi.org/10.1093/ofid/ofx146.

Smith, Tara C., and Dorit Rubinstein Reiss. "Digging the Rabbit Hole, COVID-19 Edition: Anti-vaccine Themes and the Discourse around COVID-19." *Microbes and Infection* 22, no. 10 (November-December 2020): 608–10. https://doi.org/10.1016/j.micinf.2020.11.001.

Rosselli, R., M. Martini, and N. L. Bragazzi. "The Old and the New: Vaccine Hesitancy in the Era of the Web 2.0. Challenges and Opportunities." *Journal of Preventive Medicine and Hygiene* 57, no. 1 (March 1, 2016): E47–50. https://www.ncbi.nlm.nih.gov/pmc/articles/PMC4910443/.

Boylston, Arthur W. "The Origins of Inoculation." *Journal of the Royal Society of Medicine* 105, no. 7 (July 28, 2012): 309–13. https://doi.org/10.1258/ jrsm.2012.12k044.

Larson, Heidi, Emmanuela Gakidou, and Christopher J. L. Murray. "The Vaccine-Hesitant Moment." *The New England Journal of Medicine* 387, no. 1 (July 7, 2022): 58–65. https://doi.org/10.1056/nejmra2106441.

Harvey, Amanda M., Sharlynn Thompson, Andrew Lac, and Frederick L. Coolidge. "Fear and Derision: A Quantitative Content Analysis of Provaccine and Antivaccine Internet Memes." *Health Education & Behavior* 46, no. 6 (September 6, 2019): 1012–23. https://doi.org/10.1177/10901981 19866886.

Bajaj, Simar S., and Fatima Cody Stanford. "Beyond Tuskegee—Vaccine Distrust and Everyday Racism." *The New England Journal of Medicine* 384, no. 5 (February 4, 2021): e12. https://doi.org/10.1056/nejmpv2035827.

Green, Alex. "Going Viral in the Online Anti-Vaccine Wars." *Wellcome Collection*, December 7, 2017. https://wellcomecollection.org/articles/Whf_ BSkAACsAgwil.

Tomori, Cecília, Aziza Ahmed, Dabney P. Evans, Benjamin Mason Meier, and Aparna Nair. "Your Health Is in Your Hands? US CDC COVID-

19 Mask Guidance Reveals the Moral Foundations of Public Health." *EClinicalMedicine* 38 (August 9, 2021): 101071. https://doi.org/10.1016/j.eclinm.2021.101071.

Gozzi, Nicolò, Matteo Chinazzi, Natalie E. Dean, Ira M. Longini Jr., M. Elizabeth Halloran, Nicola Perra, and Alessandro Vespignani. "Estimating the Impact of COVID-19 Vaccine Inequities: A Modeling Study." *Nature Communications* 14, no. 1 (June 6, 2023). https://doi.org/10.1038/s41467-023-39098-w.

Lazarus, Jeffrey V., Salim S. Abdool Karim, Carolina Batista, Kenneth Rabin, and Ayman El-Mohandes. "Vaccine Inequity and Hesitancy Persist— We Must Tackle Both." *BMJ*, January 3, 2023: 8. https://doi.org/10.1136/bmj.p8.

CDC. "Role of the Advisory Committee on Immunization Practices in CDC's Vaccine Recommendations." *Centers for Disease Control and Prevention.* Accessed September 18, 2023. https://www.cdc.gov/vaccines/acip/committee/role-vaccine-recommendations.html.

Bernstein, Alison. "Ask SciMoms: Where Does the Vaccine Schedule Come From?" *SciMoms*, March 5, 2019.

CDC. "Recommended Vaccines by Disease." Vaccines and Preventable Diseases, *Centers for Disease Control and Prevention.* Accessed September 18, 2023. https://www.cdc.gov/vaccines/vpd/vaccines-diseases.html.

Offit, Paul A. "Thimerosal and Vaccines—A Cautionary Tale." *The New England Journal of Medicine* 357, no. 13 (September 27, 2007): 1278–79. https://doi.org/10.1056/nejmp078187.

CDC. "Frequently Asked Questions for the Public." Hepatitis B Information, *Centers for Disease Control and Prevention.* Accessed September 18, 2023. https://www.cdc.gov/hepatitis/hbv/bfaq.htm.

ACOG. "Human Papillomavirus (HPV): Infection and Vaccination." *ACOG.* Accessed September 18, 2023. https://www.acog.org/womens-health/faqs/hpv-vaccination.

"Voices for Vaccines." Accessed September 18, 2023. https://www.voices-forvaccines.org/.

"Immunizations." *HealthyChildren.org.* Accessed September 18, 2023. https://www.healthychildren.org/English/safety-prevention/immunizations/.

9: doing the right thing

McGough, Matt, Krutika Amin, Nirmita Panchal, and Cynthia Cox. "Child and Teen Firearm Mortality in the US and Peer Countries." *KFF*, July 18, 2023. https://www.kff.org/mental-health/issue-brief/child-and-teen-fire-arm-mortality-in-the-u-s-and-peer-countries/.

Bridge, Jeffrey A., Donna A. Ruch, Arielle H. Sheftall, Hyeouk Chris Hahm, Victoria M. O'Keefe, Cynthia A. Fontanella, Guy Brock, John V. Campo, and Lisa M. Horowitz. "Youth Suicide during the First Year of the COVID-19 Pandemic." *Pediatrics* 151, no. 3 (February 15, 2023). https://doi.org/10.1542/peds.2022-058375.

Berkowitz, Steven. "As the Mental Health Crisis in Children and Teens Worsens, the Dire Shortage of Mental Health Providers Is Preventing Young People from Getting the Help They Need." *The Conversation*, August 16, 2023. https://theconversation.com/as-the-mental-health-crisis-in-children-and-teens-worsens-the-dire-shortage-of-mental-health-providers-is-preventing-young-people-from-getting-the-help-they-need-207476.

"Safety & Prevention." *HealthyChildren.org*. Accessed September 18, 2023. https://www.healthychildren.org/English/safety-prevention/Pages/default.aspx.

Harris, Meena. "Meena Harris: Kids Can Be Ambitious without Picking a Career." *Parents*, April 15, 2023. https://www.parents.com/meena-harris-on-kids-and-ambition-7229702.

Chetty, Raj, Matthew O. Jackson, Theresa Kuchler, Johannes Stroebel, Nathaniel Hendren, Robert B. Fluegge, Sara Gong, et al. "Social Capital II: Determinants of Economic Connectedness." *Nature* 608, no. 7921 (August 1, 2022): 122–34. https://doi.org/10.1038/s41586-022-04997-3.

Index

Page numbers in *italics* indicate illustrations.

postpartum mental-health issues and, 47–48

problems with, 36, 41

exposome, 182

exposure and exposome, 178–81

F

fatness and fatphobia

    BMI and, 157, 158, 161, 162

    as choice, 156–58, 161

    defining obesity, 58

    outcomes of, 156

    parents' bodies and, 164–65

    screen time and, 155–56

Fearing the Black Body: The Racial Origins of Fat Phobia (Strings), 157

Fed Is Best Foundation, 36, 54

feminism, as intersectionality as a practice of radical inclusion, 148

flame retardants, 203–4

Flint, Michigan, 198

food

    access to, 192–93

    animal agriculture, 229–30

    best-by and sell-by dates, 230

    choosing alternatives, 194

    clean eating and, 169, 187–88

    cooking, 232–33

    corn as part of industrial complex, 236–37, 238–39

    denigration of conventionally grown food, 175

    environmental costs of, 208, 209, 227–29, 230, 231–32

    EWG's Dirty Dozen, 176, 187

    GMO, 183, 237

    milk, 231–32

    MSG and, 170–73

    organic food, 173–76

    plant-based meat industry and, 231

    systemic changes to change outcomes, 169, 237–39

Ford, Donna Y., 53

formula feeding

    capitalism and, 39–41

    as costly, 34–35

    as harmful, 34–35, 42–43, 44

    studies of, 47

    supplementing breastfeeding with, 51–52, 56

    with unregulated homemade formula, 194

Foundation for Black Women's Wellness (FFBWW), 109

Fowler, Lauren A., 160

Fulton, Kari, 222

fundamental attribution error (FAE), 18–19

furry protocol rumors, 57–59

G

Gates, Bill, 20, 21

gay individuals as pedophiles, 60

GDP data, 21

Gelembiuk, Greg, 113–14

gender

    as binary, 64–65, 67–68

    bone density and, 69

    definition of, 61–62